POSITIVELY PARKINSON'S

of related interest

Can I tell you about Parkinson's Disease?
A guide for family, friends and carers
Alan M. Hultquist
ISBN 978 1 84905 948 0
eISBN 978 0 85700 767 4

Positively Parkinson's

Symptoms and Diagnosis,
Research and Treatment,
Advice and Support

Ann Andrews

Jessica Kingsley *Publishers*
London and Philadelphia

First published in 2011 by Calico Publishing Ltd.
This edition published in 2013
by Jessica Kingsley Publishers
116 Pentonville Road
London N1 9JB, UK
by arrangement with Calico Publishing

www.jkp.com

Text copyright © Ann Andrews
Illustrations © Calico Publishing Ltd
Foreword copyright © Dr Barry Snow

Library of Congress Cataloging in Publication Data
A CIP catalog record for this book is available from the Library of Congress

British Library Cataloguing in Publication Data
A CIP catalogue record for this book is available from the British Library

ISBN 978 1 84905 411 9

Printed and bound in Great Britain

*To my friends with Parkinson's who shared their
experiences so that others might benefit*

Contents

Foreword

There is a saying in Parkinson's disease medicine that when you have seen one person with Parkinson's disease, you have seen one person with Parkinson's disease. Parkinson's is a complex and intensely personal disease. Each person, patient, carer or health professional is affected in different ways, and each person has a story to tell. I have been working now for 25 years with people with Parkinson's disease, and not a week goes by when I don't learn something new. I am repeatedly reminded that each person has a unique version of the disease.

There is so much to learn and so much to know about living with the condition. There is also a bewildering amount of information in books and on the internet. Much of this information is impersonal, clinical and of uncertain relevance to someone coming to terms with their own version of a variable condition.

Ann has her own story of Parkinson's, and here she has also gathered the stories of others. Each is important, each is relevant and each deserves to be heard. My congratulations to Ann for taking on this task. I hope everyone values reading this book as much as I have.

Dr Barry Snow, Neurologist
MBChB, FRACP, FRCPC

ACKNOWLEDGEMENTS

I am grateful to those at the Centre for Brain Research at the University of Auckland who have helped me better understand the complexities of the Parkinson brain, in particular to its director, Professor Richard Faull, for allowing me such free access to his staff; to Associate Professor Bronwen Connor, for patiently teaching me about stem cells and for cross-checking my material; to Associate Professor Debbie Young, for her explanation of gene therapy; to Dr Cathy Stinear, for explaining neural plasticity; to Dr Henry Waldvogel, for his advice on anatomy; and to Laura Fogg, the centre's manager, for her direction and advice.

Special thanks to neurologist Dr Barry Snow, Honorary Clinical Associate Professor at the University of Auckland's School of Medicine, for encouraging and endorsing this project from concept to print.

My thanks also to movement clinic nurse Lorraine McDonald, for always being accessible and enthusiastic, and to my Parkinson's field officer Kay McGarry, for her practical advice. I am grateful for the support from Parkinson's New Zealand and to CEO Deirdre O'Sullivan.

Warmest thanks to my friend, physiotherapist Dinah Bradley, for her many expressions of support and permission to use her material on breathing; and to speech therapist, Jeanette Gillibrand, who diligently put me through the Lee Silverman Voice Treatment course. Thanks also to dental hygienist Corinne Boes, for her dental care guidance; Barbs Baird, for her yoga exercises; and my doctor Christine Forster, for caring for me throughout.

Thanks are also due to occupational therapist Tracey Harrington; Geraint Phillips, Therapeutics Clinic Director, Department of

Optometry and Vision Science, University of Auckland; music therapist Alison Cooper; lawyer Brian Gubb; finance advisor Murray Weatherston; and dancer John Heginbotham.

Thank you also to my editor and publisher Linda Cassells for having such faith in me and my writing, and to Sir John Walker for his participation and enthusiastic endorsement of the finished manuscript. My gratitude to Max Ritchie and Sue Giddens from the Neurological Foundation of New Zealand for their wholehearted support and endorsement, and to the David Levene Foundation for its unconditional generosity.

Last but not least, I would like to acknowledge my friends and colleagues, members of the Auckland Parkinson's Society and contributors to this book who have shared their own experiences of Parkinson's so generously: Dale Armstrong; Leslie Arnold; Cathy Christie; Robyn Egan; Christine Hayter; Roger and Glenis Hicks; Michael Jaffe; Pat Malloy; Judith Meaken; David and Anne Murrell; Maurice and Karen Nicholson; Kathy Pilbrow; Chandra Raniga; Warwick Roger; David Schafer; Raewyn Thorburn; and Don and Margie Woodward.

To my family who continue to share my journey – all my love.

Introduction

This book is written for people like me who have Parkinson's, and for our families, friends, doctors and those working in the field. It began as a wish to share everything I've learned about Parkinson's since diagnosis nearly 12 years ago. It is still the book I wish I'd had when first diagnosed, though it now contains information that you might not need till later. In this way it has become relevant to a much wider group. I see it as a book to be read through and then dipped into as the need arises.

What you will find here is a record of my own and others' experience of living with Parkinson's. It has been an opportunity for us to pass on to those of you newly diagnosed, and to your family and friends, something of what we have learned.

Over a series of informal get-togethers a group of us with Parkinson's realised we'd all had similar experiences after our initial diagnosis. Eager to learn as much as possible, we'd searched the internet and local libraries only to find that much of the information was gloomy and depressing. We already felt depressed about the uncertainty of our future with this condition, and the material we read made us feel worse.

Most of us were diagnosed some years ago, and we have now reached a point where we would like to share some of our knowledge and experience, and to provide something more individual, less clinical, and hopefully more reassuring than what we first read.

So here it is. This book is meant for you, the one with Parkinson's. And you're not alone. There are a lot of us going through a similar experience to yours. We hope that by the time you've finished reading this book you'll want to share it with family and friends, so they too have a better understanding of Parkinson's. At the very least they might come to understand that Parkinson's is not just a tremor disease, but something much more complicated.

Everyone experiences Parkinson's differently. The treatment that works for one may not work for another, as you will see from the personal stories included in this book. What we all have in common, however, is the language of Parkinson's. Like any illness, it has its own vocabulary. You've probably already come across some new words like 'levodopa', 'dyskinesia' and 'dopamine'. All these terms and many others are dealt with in the chapters ahead, but you'll also find them in the glossary at the end of this book. If the terms seem daunting at first, don't worry. You have the rest of your life to get to know them.

You won't need to know everything about Parkinson's for some time, and what you do find out won't all necessarily apply to you. In the beginning you'll be extremely sensitive to each new symptom that comes along. Now, when I read back through my notes, I'm embarrassed to see how I recorded each small anxiety.

Symptoms change over time. The little tic in the big toe of my right foot has gone. The toe now wriggles up and down and the toes on my left foot clench – I've no idea what they might do next.

The most useful suggestion I can make is that if you are fortunate enough to live near a Parkinson's Society or Parkinsonism Society, get in touch with them. (There is no real difference between these two names, except that a Parkinsonism Society represents everyone who suffers from any form of Parkinson's-like illness.) If there is no local branch, look for a national Parkinson's organisation through the internet. They all have websites.

Most importantly, do as much as you can to take responsibility for your own situation. When I look at the stories of the men and women who have shared their stories here, I'm reminded of how we've all learned to adapt to our condition. We have acquired a medical team we can trust, joined a society that is there to help us, and accessed advice, tuition and information through a range of health and fitness resources. We've been making the best of our situation, just getting on with Parkinson's. I hope this book helps you do the same.

CHAPTER 1

---◦◦◦◦◦---

What Is Parkinson's?

What is Parkinson's? This is the first question you wish you'd remembered to ask at the time of diagnosis. Even if you were told, you probably can't remember what your doctor said.

Parkinson's is a progressive disease of the brain that affects the nervous system. It is a mystery illness in many ways. It began long before you were aware you had it. In most cases, there is no known cause, and as yet there is no cure. Its progress is slow and it will alter your life, but it will not kill you.

An illness with no obvious cause is described as 'idiopathic'. Your family doctor or neurologist may refer to your illness as 'idiopathic Parkinson's', which simply means they don't know what has caused the disease. One of the reasons why I think of Parkinson's as a mystery illness is that the diagnosis requires no blood test, no x-ray, no poking and prodding – just an observation and a chat. From the point of diagnosis onwards your medical care will mostly continue in this manner, through observation and discussion.

Another mystery of Parkinson's is that no two people seem to get it in the same way. For instance, you may be prescribed medication at an earlier or later stage than someone else; it will be a different combination of drugs from theirs; and you may have a different response. This can sometimes make treatment seem like trial and error.

Although in most cases there is no absolute cause of Parkinson's, we do know that it results from a loss of neurons that produce dopamine, an important chemical messenger in the brain that helps initiate movement. We don't know why this loss occurs. The main area in the brain where these dopamine-producing neurons are lost is called the substantia nigra. I've an idea of roughly where in the brain this is, but I've never needed to know more about the substantia nigra than that it gets its name from being blackish in colour, and is involved in a variety of brain functions such as voluntary movements, spatial awareness and mood regulation.

In researching this book, I've looked at the brain more closely than I'd ever done before. As a result, I have a slightly better understanding of its complexities. At the same time, I am more aware of the calamities that can occur when something goes wrong.

The brain contains areas specialising in independent tasks, yet somehow these areas are synchronised to maintain us as the person we have come to know and trust. When one of the areas in our brain is damaged or destroyed after an accident, stroke or haemorrhage, the result is abrupt disorder and a loss of capacity that can tragically change forever the individual we are.

In Parkinson's, the loss of dopamine in the substantia nigra doesn't cause an immediate or dramatic change, as in the case of a stroke. Instead, over time you slowly lose the ability to do things you previously took for granted. The effect is most noticeable in movement, which is why Parkinson's is also called a movement disorder, and why you may be referred to a movement clinic.

By the time you've been referred to such a specialist clinic, you will have developed one of the four main symptoms that characterise Parkinson's: tremor; bradykinesia or slowing of movement; stiffness and rigidity; and loss of balance. One of the first things you will have noticed is that the symptom is on one side of your body only. This is intriguing. Why only on one side, and why that particular side? Is it anything to do with being left- or right-handed? Probably not, as symptoms often appear on the opposite side to the dominant one. It is just another of Parkinson's mysteries. Most of us continue to feel that one side of our body is more affected than the other, even after a number of years when cell loss may be occurring on both sides of the brain.

What causes Parkinson's?

The cause of Parkinson's remains unknown, but because it is human nature to want to have a reason for everything, it's natural to search for the answer ourselves. We think there has to be something – some event in the past, something we ingested, somewhere we lived, some work we did, an injury we had, a virus we caught. Perhaps we have inherited a gene that has a predisposition to Parkinson's, and something has happened to trigger this gene into action. Some of you may even remember a parent or close relative who had Parkinson's, but there are only a small number of families where hereditary Parkinson's has been absolutely identified. There is no history of it in my family.

Some tranquillisers and other drugs have been known to cause Parkinson's symptoms, but these are usually reversible once the medication is ceased. However, in the early 1980s Stanford University scientists discovered that an illicit drug called MPTP, produced accidentally during the manufacture of another synthetic opioid drug called MPPP, was the cause of irreversible Parkinson's symptoms. When drug addict George Carillo took MPTP-contaminated heroin, the effect was almost instantaneous final-stage Parkinson's. The drug had catastrophically destroyed nerve cells, leaving him frozen and mute, locked in by his own body. (The case is described in *The Case of the Frozen Addicts* by Dr J. William Langston and in a *Time* magazine article by Claudia Wallis, 'Surprising Clue to Parkinson's'.)

When I read this story I couldn't help thinking about an experience I had in my late thirties. A friend who grew his own marijuana offered me a smoke. I took just two puffs and over the next few minutes began to feel extremely dizzy and had to lie down. Soon I was mute and paralysed, though still able to think, hear and see. It was absolutely terrifying, like being buried alive. I feared I would stay like that forever, trapped in a body that was no longer able to communicate that it was still conscious.

I don't remember how long it lasted; it may have been anything from five to 20 minutes. It felt longer. Once I began to be able to move, everything quickly returned to normal. I seemed to suffer no long-term effect, but the event was so frightening that I never smoked dope again. Until I read the account of George Carillo, I hadn't even considered a connection between that experience and my development of Parkinson's. Could this have been the trigger in my case?

I also spent my childhood living in a rural area where DDT and other pesticides were used. I worked in market gardens and orchards during holidays at a time when sprays were applied freely without the precaution of a mask or protective clothing. Once in my own garden I discovered a tree stripped of its leaves by hundreds of brown caterpillars. I took one of the caterpillars to the local garden centre and was advised which insecticide I'd need. I went home, put on some overalls and tied a scarf cowboy-style around my face, mixed up the spray and sprayed the tree. There was a slight breeze and some of the spray blew back onto me. That night and the next day I felt nauseous. The caterpillars died and the tree lived on, but what about me? Was that spraying session the trigger for my Parkinson's?

One of the men I interviewed for this book felt there could be a connection between spinal damage and Parkinson's. He had been treated for severe back pain for quite some time before being diagnosed with Parkinson's. A number of others, including myself, suffered from severe back pain before we were diagnosed.

Another of the men I spoke to wondered whether his Parkinson's was caused by the variety of solvents containing toxic substances that he is exposed to in his work. Others have blamed pesticides, herbicides and dioxins such as Agent Orange. Scientists have studied viruses for links. Former world heavyweight boxing champion Muhammad Ali has Parkinson's, but whether he got it from boxing is debatable.

What we can agree on is that we don't yet know what causes Parkinson's, even though a lot of money is being spent trying to find out. All we can be sure of is that Parkinson's results from a loss of dopaminergic neurons in the brain.

Dopamine

Dopaminergic neurons are nerve cells that release the chemical neurotransmitter dopamine. The dopamine remains in the nerve terminals of the cells until electrical impulses release it to target cells that facilitate movement. In this way, dopamine is largely responsible for motor control – for coordinating muscles so that we move smoothly and quickly. It also helps regulate our mood. When the ability to produce dopamine is reduced to the point where about 80 per cent of the dopamine cells in the brain are lost, the symptoms of Parkinson's appear.

Movement areas of the brain

One way the brain makes us move:

1. The executive function part of the cerebral cortex plans the move.

2. The substantia nigra produces dopamine and facilitates the basal ganglia to control the move.

3. The basal ganglia instructs the motor cortex to make the move. The basal ganglia (shown shaded in the cross-section below) is a cluster of nuclei: the caudate nucleus, thalamus, globus pallidus and the substantia nigra.

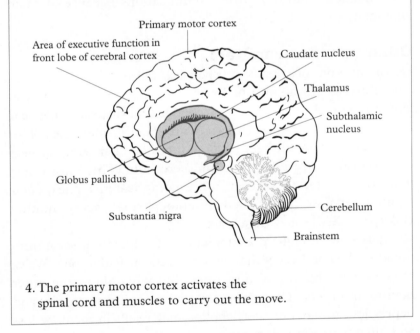

Primary motor cortex

Area of executive function in front lobe of cerebral cortex

Caudate nucleus

Thalamus

Subthalamic nucleus

Globus pallidus

Substantia nigra

Cerebellum

Brainstem

4. The primary motor cortex activates the spinal cord and muscles to carry out the move.

We now know dopamine-producing cells are also to be found in the gut and the intestines, and that there is a deficiency of intestinal dopamine cells in people with Parkinson's. This seems to indicate that Parkinson's is not just a condition affecting the dopamine in the substantia nigra. Some people with Parkinson's do experience varying gastrointestinal symptoms, but the role of dopamine in the gut is not yet clear.

Since it was discovered in 1967, a medication called levodopa has remained the predominant method of treatment for Parkinson's. Levodopa (marketed under the trade names of Sinemet and Madopar) converts into dopamine once it reaches the substantia nigra. Levodopa doesn't treat the underlying cause of the dopamine deficiency; it supplements the remaining dopamine enough to control the symptoms. It is only effective in aiding motor function.

When it was first trialled levodopa caused nausea. The drug carbidopa was then added; it prevents nausea, but also helps more levodopa cross the blood–brain barrier so that less is required to ensure a successful treatment. Prior to the development of levodopa, most people with Parkinson's were immobilised for five to 15 years after diagnosis and died from complications because of their immobility.

Other neurotransmitters

Dopamine is one of a number of chemicals called neurotransmitters. These are chemicals in our brain that carry messages across neurons, a bit like an internet provider, except that each chemical or neurotransmitter carries its own specific messages. The neurotransmitters you will become more familiar with because of Parkinson's are dopamine and serotonin. There are other neurotransmitters with even more complicated names, such as noradrenaline (also called norepinephrine), acetylcholine, endorphin, GABA and glutamate.

It is now thought that depletion of dopamine, serotonin, noradrenaline and acetylcholine may occur in Parkinson's. We've talked about the loss of dopamine, but what about the other neurotransmitters? The loss of serotonin may cause anxiety and depression; the loss of acetylcholine may result in memory loss and affect nerve impulses to the heart, brain, muscles, stomach and bladder; the loss of noradrenaline may affect the autonomic nervous system.

The autonomic nervous system (ANS)

Unless you're a scientist or medical professional, you probably haven't heard of the autonomic nervous system, or ANS, before. However, those of us with Parkinson's will get to know it well. As Parkinson's progresses, the degenerative process extends beyond the substantia nigra to the hypothalamus; the hypothalamus is where the ANS begins, extending via the spinal cord through the nervous system to the vital organs that regulate the body's involuntary activities. The ANS regulates:

+ The organs:
    - heart
    - lungs
    - brain
    - stomach, intestines and bladder
    - liver
    - kidneys
    - skin
    - eyes
    - blood vessels.

+ The glands:
    - oral/nasal mucosa
    - salivary
    - adrenals.

The ANS has three divisions: the sympathetic system, the parasympathetic system and the enteric system. Two of these systems are affected by Parkinson's: the sympathetic and the parasympathetic. These two work in tandem, but often in opposition. The sympathetic system leaps in when you need an immediate response (as in an emergency) by raising your blood pressure and increasing your heart rate. The parasympathetic system works at conserving energy, controlling relaxation and aiding digestion. It lowers the blood pressure and the heart rate.

The autonomic nervous system (ANS)

The hypothalamus is situated at the top of the brainstem just below the thalamus. It controls the ANS.

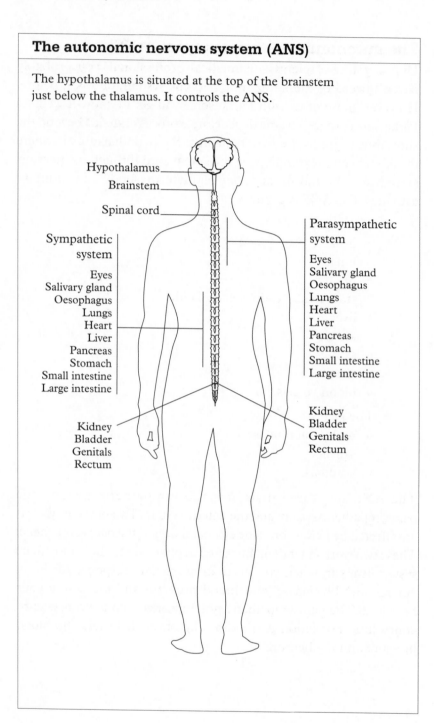

In this way the ANS controls your temperature, blood pressure, heart and respiratory rate – the vital signs that your doctor checks whenever you turn up for a consultation. It also controls the immune system, regulates your glands and the muscles of your organs and takes care of all the things you do without realising and therefore take for granted.

The effect of Parkinson's on the ANS is the less visible side of the disease. It can affect your skin, hair, eyes, perspiration, speech, saliva, swallowing, sleep and bladder control. It may cause postural hypotension when the blood pressure drops suddenly as you move from one position to another, causing dizziness, fatigue and light-headedness. It may lower your immunity, dry up your saliva to the point where you can barely talk or swallow, or it may increase perspiration to an embarrassing degree. The symptoms you experience can be so subtle as to be barely noticeable, or so bothersome that they affect your daily life. Mostly, they will be invisible to family, friends and observers accustomed to associating Parkinson's mainly with tremor and stiffness.

CHAPTER 2

Primary Symptoms and Diagnosis

The diagnosis of Parkinson's depends on finding evidence of four distinct characteristic symptoms of the disease: tremor; bradykinesia or slowing of movement; stiffness and rigidity; and loss of balance. There is no blood test, x-ray or MRI scan that identifies Parkinson's; these tests may simply help to eliminate other possible causes. Because the diagnosis is largely observational, the final verdict can be difficult to accept.

It is some years since I was diagnosed with Parkinson's. I am fit and enjoy a busy lifestyle. I didn't have all four main symptoms in the beginning, though I do now. I've drawn on my own experience as well as that of others to describe these symptoms for you. My first obvious sign of Parkinson's was a tremor, and because this is the most overt symptom, it is the one that people most often associate with the condition, although about 30 per cent of us won't have any tremor at all.

Often I'm asked what the first sign was that I had of Parkinson's, something I find difficult to answer. In retrospect, I had quite a few clues, but I do remember the first twitch. I was staying at my mother's house and had just gone to bed when my big toe twitched. I took no notice initially, but it wouldn't stop, and so I assumed it was some kind of muscle tic. It never really went away after that.

Tremor

I'm not sure how long it was before my hand started to shake, though I remember one very early occasion. My husband was out one evening. I'd gone to bed and must have been asleep for some time when I was woken by a sound from outside. I checked the clock and saw it was early morning. There was no sign of my husband, and as I began to feel anxious my hand started to shake. Of course, he was quite well and having imbibed a little too much had sensibly decided to sleep at a friend's house. As soon as he phoned and I knew all was well the tremor ceased. Now, of course, I understand that what happened to me that night was the beginning of a Parkinson's tremor. At first I mostly experienced it when anxious, but now it's with me most of the time.

Officially, it's called a 'resting tremor', as it occurs when your hand is at rest. It's described as a pill-rolling action because it can look like you're rolling a pill between your index finger and thumb. I've studied my tremor and it has never quite looked like this; it looks more like a rhythmic shake of the hand. The tremor in my leg is less vigorous, but more constant. It's a later arrival and jiggles me when I'm applying my make-up, chopping vegetables and typing on my computer.

Bradykinesia or slowing of movement

I'm just beginning to experience the slowness of movement that is bradykinesia. It's harder to switch on the lights, get dressed, tie my laces and do up my buttons. As I struggle to put shoes on my grandchildren or fasten them into their seat belts I am confronted by my loss. I'm so aware of how frustrated these babies and toddlers must feel, wanting to use hands and fingers that don't yet have the strength and dexterity to do everything they want. I empathise with their wish to do things themselves and am humbled at how patient they are to accept help from me, who is so much slower than their parents.

This newly experienced slowness causes a few problems. The act of eating requires the movement of many muscles; when these muscles slow down they can affect chewing, swallowing and the passing of food to the stomach. My problem seems to be a slow response from the muscles that seal off the windpipe and stop food or liquid from getting in. This results in fits of choking. After I'd had a series of bronchial infections, my doctor suggested a barium swallow test in case there was some serious problem. The test showed only the slowing of the muscles. So now I take smaller bites, chew food well and am more aware of how I swallow.

Occasionally, when getting out of a car I have to wait until my body moves. This difficulty in beginning a movement is called a 'start hesitation' and is another sign of bradykinesia. If this happens when I'm by myself, I can hoist on the door; if I've got company, I might ask for a push.

We made a family DVD recently of us all walking in the park and I was surprised to see the extent to which my walk had changed. I've developed a hesitation in my right leg and swing my right foot inwards. I can still consciously correct this and it doesn't stop me running when I want to.

If you are newly diagnosed, you probably won't experience any of these symptoms for quite some time. There is one aspect of bradykinesia which, thank goodness, I've still not experienced. This is an inability to complete a movement, and may be most noticeable when someone has difficulty rolling over in bed or getting up from a chair. I remember when my grandsons were only babies and couldn't yet roll over or sit up. Watching them, I was so aware of the strength they had yet to develop to accomplish these actions which later, as children and adults, we take for granted.

Stiffness and rigidity

The rigidity of Parkinson's can prevent muscles from relaxing, and the continual tension makes muscles ache. The result can be that you go to sleep with the ache of tired muscles and wake with the ache of stiff muscles. Stretching exercises are essential, and I've found doing them every morning keeps me supple.

One of the earliest symptoms of stiffness I noticed was in my right arm, which I realised one day I was holding rigid, bent at the elbow with my fist clenched at waist level. This rigidity in an arm is often described as a failure to swing the arm when walking, but once you're on medication it usually eases. The other two most described symptoms of stiffness are in the face. You may not blink as much as most people do, or your facial muscles can tighten to a degree where it becomes difficult to show any expression. This is usually referred to as 'facial masking'.

Loss of balance

This is one of the first things your doctor tests for. He or she will stand behind you and, after promising to catch you, will gently pull back on your shoulders, just like one of those exercises to develop trust. At the time it seems a strange thing to do, but loss of balance is one of the main symptoms of Parkinson's. The lack of dopamine in the brain results in the loss of the 'righting reflex'. When tipped off balance, whether by your own manoeuvring or by an external force, you'll probably find it hard to stay straight. Moving rapidly over uneven terrain is no longer possible; you become hesitant, where once you were confident, and maybe you have a few falls.

There's another phenomenon called 'retropulsion', where your body develops a tendency to fall backwards. I've only just begun to notice this. It can be a nuisance when you're trying to put your trousers on while standing. Make sure there's a wall handy to lean or fall back on. Retropulsion can be embarrassing at social functions if your backward movement is mistaken for inebriation.

Because of the slow onset of Parkinson's you may not notice all these symptoms for quite some time, and it's possible that you'll become so used to some of the changes in your body that you won't notice them until someone points them out. Once you've heard the diagnosis of Parkinson's, though, you'll remember all the small signs you've experienced over a long period of time leading up to this moment.

Diagnosis

Parkinson's is often thought of as an old person's disease. However, some of those diagnosed will be under the age of 50. They are usually described as having early-onset Parkinson's. I was 59 when diagnosed and yet my neurologist told me I had early-onset. I soon found there were quite a few others about my age also described as early-onset.

In talking to others about their experience, I found so many similarities with my own. Like me, they all went through a gamut of tests with a neurologist as part of a process of elimination. In the end, it was a series of surprisingly simple tasks that confirmed Parkinson's – walking across the room, touching your nose with your finger, and trusting the neurologist to pull you gently backwards and tip you off balance. It probably wasn't quite as basic as that, but that's how it seemed.

The neurologist who diagnosed me gave me a booklet and a prescription for the levodopa drug called Sinemet. He told me to take the medication, three tablets a day, for the next month and return for a further check. It was all very ordinary. I remember walking to my car and driving home as if nothing had happened. I didn't know what to think. I'd just been told I had a chronic illness, but it wouldn't kill me. So was that serious or not?

I read through the booklet, and after reading about side effects of the medication, I knew there was no way I wanted to take it unless I had to. At this stage the medication seemed worse than the diagnosis.

After dinner that night I told my husband. He was surprised; he'd forgotten I was even going to see a neurologist. I gave him the booklet to read. The booklet explained a lot of things about the condition, some quite scary, particularly the description of Parkinson's as progressive. It seemed to have little to do with me or my life. None of it was happening now, but like the spell the wicked witch cast on the little princess in *Sleeping Beauty* – it would happen to me some time in the future.

I made an appointment to see my doctor. Because Parkinson's strikes so few people in the community, your doctor may have little experience of caring for patients with the disease, particularly in younger people. So it may be that you and your doctor find yourselves on a joint learning curve, one armed with the theory, and the other bearing the problem. When I saw my doctor, I felt the need to express my concern about staying in the continued care of the neurologist I'd just seen. She told me I could seek a second opinion and wrote me a referral.

There was one event I observed with the first neurologist which appalled me at the time and worried me later. It happened when I was in hospital for some of the initial tests. I was in a ward with six women, all much older than me. Four of us were patients of the same neurologist. One morning he came into the ward with two registrars and discussed the other women individually quite loudly, as if they were not present. The women were in the latter stages of Parkinson's and I found it immensely sad and depressing to see them treated with such disrespect. When I learned I too had Parkinson's, I was afraid that this could happen to me as the condition progressed. I went to another neurologist and had a completely different, far more reassuring experience.

Try to find a neurologist who has undertaken further specialist training in Parkinsonism or movement disorders, and preferably one you feel you can trust and be comfortable with. You don't have to stay with the first person you see. I had about four private visits with my chosen neurologist, and then learned I could see him through the hospital system. The appointments are shorter, but at no cost, and now that I'm part of the public health system I have access to a lot more services such as physiotherapy, and occupational and speech therapy. So don't worry if you're unable to afford seeing a neurologist or therapists privately, you can access specialist treatment through your nearest hospital. But what if you can't relate to your allotted hospital neurologist? This happened to a friend of mine, and she contacted the clinic manager and was moved to another specialist for her next visit.

After the first visit you may remember little of what the neurologist told you about Parkinson's. The whole appointment may be a bit of a blur. Over the next few weeks you will no doubt think of many questions you wish you'd asked. This is usual. Write your questions down as they arise, and keep a file of them for your next visit. Then remember to take a pen or, better still, a family member prepared with a pen to write down the answers.

The accurate diagnosis of Parkinson's can be difficult in some people; their response to drugs and emerging symptoms may lead to a reassessment. The term 'Parkinsonism' covers a variety of conditions that result in involuntary movements. There are a number of similar disorders that are sometimes grouped together: these include essential tremor, a tremor that may be in the hands, arms, head, neck, jaw or voice, but occurs when making a voluntary movement rather than a resting tremor, as in Parkinson's; SWEDDs, an acronym for subjects without evidence of dopaminergic deficit, which refers to having a tremor of unknown origin without loss of dopamine and with no other Parkinson's symptoms; and progressive supranuclear palsy (PSP), a PD+ ('Parkinson's Plus') syndrome that progresses more rapidly than Parkinson's; and multiple system atrophy (MSA), where more than one system is degenerating. But don't panic – by the time you've reached diagnosis the indications will be pretty clear.

Having the diagnosis confirmed

▶ *Warwick is a journalist and was in his late forties when diagnosed with Parkinson's. Here he captures his experience when referred to a neurologist for a second opinion and diagnosis.*

At first we just chatted. He studied me keenly, but took no notes. I would later surmise that he was checking to see if I had that fixed stare that is characteristic of people with Parkinson's disease.

He took my blood pressure standing and lying, tapped my knees with a rubber dongy-knocker to see if they jumped. They jumped. He got me to rotate my wrists and move my hands to their fullest extent. He sort of arm-wrestled me and had a look into my eyes. He stood me up and grabbed me from behind. He told me to walk to the gate and back, observing that my right arm didn't swing. The whole process took about half an hour.

Then he sat me down and told me what I already knew. I had Parkinson's disease...

I got into my car and drove slowly back to the office, wondering as I headed down Victoria Avenue whether this crisp autumn morning was one of the days – like school leaving day, wedding day, job changing day, child's birth day, divorce day – on which my life would change forever.

It didn't really feel that way. It didn't feel like anything. Maybe I was numbed by the news, but I prefer to think that I was just being fatalistic, believing as I do that a certain number of bad things are bound to happen to you in your life, hopefully not too many, and there's not a thing you can do about them, so it's sensible to try to make the best of them. I was reasonably fit, my heart was still lion-like, and I'd just written a book I was proud of. I had four great kids, a loving wife, sufficient friends, a job, and money in the bank. The sun would, no doubt, still come up tomorrow. The neurologist had said no one ever died of Parkinson's. You die with it.

And yet…wasn't I a bit young to have a progressively debilitating disease? Wasn't this another of God's cruel jokes, the latest of rather too many he'd played on me and my family down the years? What would become of me? That was the big question…and a silly one too when you think about it, because no one knows what will become of them.

Back in the office I told a few people. They were solicitous, kind and, I have to say, for the most part ignorant about just what Parkinson's is and how it affects people who have it. Why weren't my hands shaking, they asked. Would I be able to go on working? What about my beloved cricket?

…I find it very difficult to write about the reaction of my wife to the news. Robyn is relentlessly positive about everything, whereas I have become more negative over the years. We're fundamentally very different, and I am older. Her attitude to what I was now telling her was immediate . . . and relentlessly positive: this was no big deal, we'll find out all we can about it and then we'll take a mental cold shower and beat it by sheer willpower. I took the view that it might not be that easy. Thus we had, right from the start, a clash of ideas, a difference of approach. And I think we still do.

Eleven years after Warwick's diagnosis, his father-in-law died. He had had Parkinson's for the last ten years of his life, then had a stroke which seemed to ratchet up the Parkinson's symptoms. No longer able to care for himself, he required 24-hour hospital care. His father-in-law's illness and subsequent death had a profound effect on Warwick, who has since developed severe dyskinesia – that is, an increase in involuntary movements and less control over voluntary movements. What Warwick faced as he watched his father-in-law's deterioration was the very thing he had been most afraid of since being told at the time of his diagnosis that Parkinson's was a progressive disease.

The Shorter Oxford Dictionary *defines progressive disease as 'continuously increasing in severity or extent'. But how severe, and to what extent, and increasing how quickly? There's the rub. In Warwick's words: 'Who is to know how quickly, or how slowly, it will progress? We only know that it will.'*

Warwick stayed with the neurologist he originally saw, but others, like me, have felt less confident and moved to see someone else. This was the case for Clare.

Changing neurologists

▶ *Clare was in her mid-forties when she was diagnosed. She was a successful business woman working as a chartered accountant for a multinational company. She was told she had akinetic hemiplegic Parkinson's disease, which means she had no tremor, and the disease presented on one side only. The diagnosis shocked her. She says she got the fright of her life, but she was also unhappy with the attitude of the neurologist.*

I had no idea what the diagnosis meant for me. The neurologist was not particularly informative, and when I asked about websites, replied that they were often unreliable, but didn't advise me of any that would give me the reliable information I craved. The standard booklet he gave me was his last one, so he asked for it to be returned. I smiled meekly and agreed, knowing that I had no intention of letting go of the only information I had.

I asked about alternative therapies, as I wasn't keen on taking medication for the rest of my life. His reply was to liken it to having diabetes and always having to take insulin. The way he seemed to put it was that if I took the medication like a good compliant patient, I would be rewarded with 50 per cent better mobility for the next five years. I thought, what the hell happens after that? He did at least reassure me that I would die with Parkinson's but not from it. Small comfort!

He prescribed levodopa and within half an hour of the first dose my left knee locked, making movement more difficult than before. I was stranded in my office until the effects wore off. The next medication he prescribed made me feel 'spaced out'.

Losing confidence in him, I got a referral to another neurologist, who started me on amantadine [also known as Symmetrel], a drug originally designed to combat flu symptoms, but which also helps people with Parkinson's. It didn't improve mobility the estimated 50 per cent, but at least there were no obvious side effects. With some relief, I at last felt there was a line of communication between me and this new neurologist.

Changing neurologists restored Clare's confidence in the care she was receiving. But having confirmation of the diagnosis can unleash a whole range of varying emotions, from denial to outright rage and anger.

Shock and anger at the diagnosis

▶ *Kathy is married with two children and six grandchildren and was diagnosed with Parkinson's at the age of 60. At first she refused to find out anything more about the disease, but then she shocked her family by raging about her fear and anger.*

My doctor referred me to a physician, a kindly man. After a series of strange tests he sat forward and looked at me. Oh goodness, I thought, surely it's not anything serious? 'The tests,' he said, 'show that you may have Parkinson's.'

As he talked, the shock hit me. I pressed my eyes to stop the tears. Why hadn't I brought my husband with me? What way will it affect me? Will the family cope? Does that mean I'll die early? So many questions whirled around my brain. I had no idea what Parkinson's was. My physician recommended that I not read about it for the moment and give myself time to absorb the diagnosis with my family around me.

It took about a week before I wanted to find out about Parkinson's. All my family had checked the internet and were waiting for me to talk about it. They were shocked and concerned as they listened to me ranting on about my fears, my depression and my venting anger. I thought back over the last weeks.

I had definitely been feeling tired. I'd had an operation on my lower back a few months previously, and was still recovering from that. During that time my family helped in the way family does. I know they will always be with me, helping me when my stubbornness allows it, but with this disease I felt alone and I needed to talk to other sufferers to see how they coped. I searched the internet and discovered there are Parkinson's societies in all countries. I got in touch with my local one, and it was so worthwhile! A field officer [similar to a social worker or specialist nurse] visited and almost immediately I found that there existed support groups and meetings.

It took a while, but finally I felt I could cope with things that had been a burden. My dream of travelling to England to be with my daughter and family became a reality. That trip brought my confidence back. Flying across half the world by myself, I was able to get back most of my independence and prove I could still do the things I was able to do before Parkinson's.

▶ *For Michael, aged 66, the diagnosis was even more shocking because he had experienced Parkinson's before through the suffering of his mother. He has had to dig deep to find the courage to face it himself.*

Three years ago I noticed I had begun to drag my right foot when walking. I seemed to be slowing down and was tired by the end of each day. My shoulders and forearm were stiff and felt tight, my writing had become a scrawl and I had difficulty completing a sentence. My voice had quietened off considerably; my face looked blank at times and I had a mild tremor in my right hand. With these symptoms I went to see my physician, who after examining me advised that I had Parkinson's. The diagnosis was then confirmed by a neurologist.

How did I feel about this sudden change in my life? Understandably, I was very emotional. My family were stunned by the diagnosis. There were lots of tears and I had a sense of dread and fear that I would end up like my late mother, who died aged 81 with Parkinson's. She spent the last years of her life in a vegetative state requiring 24-hour care. I had to deal with this fear and convince myself that I would not end up like her.

Thus began an intense campaign at the very centre of my emotions. How was I to accept that life will never be the same, that I am in the honeymoon period of Parkinson's and don't know how long this period will last? Then what will happen to me? Will I become dependent on my wife to care for me? And how will she deal with this change?

Deep down inside me I know I cannot reverse this path and I am scared. Yes, I am scared in every sense of the word; scared that I may not be able to fend for myself, that I will have to be fed, toileted and washed, and I have to accept that this is the way it's going to be. Now three years on I notice subtle changes. Shaving is getting harder, fatigue at the end of the day is real, writing is a problem, and driving for more than an hour is simply not possible. The amount of medication I take and what it is doing to my system worries me, especially when I wake at 3.00 a.m. and cannot get back to sleep. Some days it takes all my determination and courage to push on.

We all respond to the diagnosis of Parkinson's in different ways, depending on our previous knowledge of it and on our personality. What dominates our thoughts is 'How bad will it get?' The path of

Parkinson's for each of us from here on is unknown. For me, the scariest unknown is what will happen as I grow older. Some of us develop dementia, but so do many people who don't even have Parkinson's. The priority for all of us is to make the most of life now.

CHAPTER 3

Early-onset Parkinson's

Although Parkinson's is usually associated with the elderly, younger people are increasingly being diagnosed with the disease. 'Early-onset Parkinson's' is the term used when the diagnosis occurs in those under the age of 50. There is now more awareness of early-onset Parkinson's, especially since international publicity around some younger, high-profile individuals such as actor Michael J. Fox, who was diagnosed at the age of 28, and Olympic champion John Walker, who was diagnosed at 43.

Parkinson's is an unpredictable disease; secondary symptoms can occur early on or after many years, and can progress at a fast or slow pace, no matter what your age. In early-onset Parkinson's, secondary symptoms seem to appear more slowly.

Although I was diagnosed in my fifties, I realise now that I had indications of Parkinson's in my late forties. The symptoms began as strange aches in my legs and my right arm, uncomfortable enough to prevent me getting to sleep at night. The aches in my legs, which I still get, are called 'restless legs' or akathisia. The ache in my arm was the beginning of a similar pain that still prompts me to sleep with my right arm held straight by my side.

These aches and pains bothered me, but I never suspected they might be symptoms of Parkinson's. Then I started having problems with vertical double vision, particularly when walking. This manifested as if people walking towards me had two heads, one on top of the other. On the road I'd see two cars, one carrying the other. If I shut one eye everything appeared normal. It was so disconcerting I didn't mention it to anyone.

Not long after this I had a coronary scare; tests showed I had coronary artery disease. I blamed the double vision on my heart problems, but even after successful coronary artery treatment the double vision persisted. I discussed it with my heart physician and my doctor. They had no idea what might be wrong and could see no connection. Today what triggered this problem remains uncertain, but it seems to be caused by a long-standing fourth nerve palsy in my left eye. One of the symptoms of Parkinson's is impairment of eye movements, but whether this could result in damage of this kind no one seems to know.

As a result of this succession of small difficulties I began to lose confidence. I had a few falls and lost the sure-footedness that I had always enjoyed when hiking or walking. I blamed this on my double vision. Later my handwriting began to deteriorate, becoming smaller and more difficult to execute. This was frustrating and embarrassing.

It must have been a couple of years later that I began to have difficulty with my speech – mostly a softening of my voice and a need to clear my throat. I would go to say something and could only manage a voice so faint and husky that people couldn't hear me. At first I felt I was being ignored. Then I hoped I hadn't been heard, as I was embarrassed at having such a small voice. Finally, I began to wonder whether I had anything to say anyway, which slowly led to feelings of complete inadequacy in meetings or on social occasions.

As one symptom followed another, my confidence continued to erode. One day I noticed I was holding my right arm rigidly at waist height. At the time, we were painting our house and I assumed that my arm was stiff from too much sanding and painting.

Finally, about ten years after those first night-time aches I developed a tremor. I went through a gamut of tests over the next months, including a lumbar puncture and an MRI. It was at the end of that year I finally learned I had Parkinson's.

That was the slow onset of Parkinson's for me. You will see from reading the experiences of others that the symptoms and progression rate vary hugely. About three quarters of us might develop an early tremor; others may never experience one, or develop it much later. However, those with the more visible tremor probably present earlier for diagnosis than those with less obvious symptoms. For those with tremor and an early diagnosis, it may seem that progression is slow, whereas for those without tremor, and perhaps a later diagnosis, progression might appear to be faster.

The onset doesn't speed up with diagnosis. In my case, over a 12-year period Parkinson's is still taking its time.

Diagnosed at the age of 44

▶ *Don's experience of Parkinson's began 20 years ago. He is 61 and was diagnosed with Parkinson's in his mid-forties. This is part of his story that he put into a small self-help booklet on his experience.*

I was 44 when diagnosed with Parkinson's. The neurologist gave me the old, 'Well, there's good and bad news' line. 'The bad news is that you have Parkinson's; the good news is that of all neurological disorders, researchers are making the most headway with Parkinson's.'

The news didn't come as too big a shock as I'd had a sneaking suspicion for the previous two years that Parkinson's was prowling round. Both my mother and her mother had suffered from it.

On the way home I thought to myself, 'Well, that's a bit of a bummer.' But I am an eternal optimist and after a few miles I thought, 'You know, if I died tomorrow, I would be in credit because I've had a fantastic life.'

One thing that I'm very grateful for is that almost without exception our friends are positive people. They say I have a marvellous attitude. Maybe I have, but I'm sure it's one of the main reasons why nearly 20 years after being diagnosed I'm on the same dose of medication and have only deteriorated marginally. In fact, it's hard to tell whether it is deterioration because of the Parkinson's or deterioration because of natural ageing.

It all started with the typical symptoms: difficulty tying shoe laces, doing up buttons, brushing my teeth and writing – although I must admit my handwriting has always been shocking. Other symptoms were a wooden facial expression, and not swinging my arms when walking. Initially, I put the symptoms down to work pressure, but what used to really wind me up was when we were at social functions and after a couple of drinks my wife would sidle up and elbow me in the ribs. 'You're drinking too much. Your speech is getting slurred.'

Fortunately for me, the prescribed medication didn't cause any side effects. Initially, I had 'switch-off' times, as though someone had flicked off the switch, and I would experience crushing tiredness. My pulse rate dropped to the mid-fifties and I felt as though all my systems had been shut down. But I would grind away and work my way through it and an hour later I'd be fine. The only other effect has been interrupted sleep. I don't mind waking at two in the morning and have come up with some brilliant ideas in what I call my most creative time of the day, but my wife gets paranoid if she doesn't get eight hours' undisturbed sleep. She also has to wake me when I'm having the vivid dreams I get from levodopa.

I don't do a lot to stay fit now, but purely by chance I got involved in masters rowing about the same time that I was diagnosed with Parkinson's. Later I met a student studying rehabilitation for stroke patients who said that rowing was beneficial because the action required the rower to use their limbs in unison. My own theory has been that if researchers come up with a cure for Parkinson's I want to be in the best possible shape to take advantage of it.

It is ten years since I first wrote about living with Parkinson's and I know that I was a bit gung-ho at the time and advocated a keep-fit-and-be-like-me philosophy. I have since met many people with Parkinson's and am aware that it comes in various forms and degrees of seriousness. I am extremely lucky that I seem to have a strain that is not deteriorating very much and the medication works well for me. But I am convinced that exercising and having a positive attitude does help. Get on with life, enjoy yourself and above all help others. The ball's in your court.

Early signs and slow development

▶ *Dale is 56, divorced, and a mother of five adult children. She was diagnosed with Parkinson's 15 years ago.*

Dale's first symptoms appeared in her thirties and began with a painful hip, tight hamstring, stiff shoulder with poor rotation, difficulty getting toes into sandals, tripping, circling hand movements and toes curling – all this on her left side.

A keen sportswoman, she put most of her symptoms down to sports injuries. However, one day when she was picking beans in her garden and her hand simply couldn't put them into her pocket, she began to think something wasn't right.

Initially, she didn't have a noticeable tremor; she was more aware of it as an internal feeling. Her tremor is now quite pronounced, especially when she is stressed or excited. Parkinson's now affects both sides of her body. She gets more dyskinesia, which gives her what she calls the 'drunken staggers'. Gardening is no longer easy or enjoyable because of loss of balance, though she feels better outside where she has the space around her to move.

Stiffness and slowness can be a problem when her medication is low. Dale feels pleased to live at a time when levodopa is available, even if she has to cope with dyskinesia.

She tires easily, and being of strong character she refuses to give in and pushes herself to do as much as possible. In the last two or three years she has been on an outdoor pursuits course and taken part in round-the-island races on the large island where she lives. She moved there some time ago and finds the relaxed way of life is sympathetic to her illness.

Her general health is pretty good, though she has lost bone density and her eyesight has deteriorated, both of which she puts down to her age. The pain she originally felt in her hip is less of a problem, but she feels frustrated by her lack of fitness. She hasn't felt anxious or depressed and certainly doesn't feel sorry for herself. As she says, 'What will be, will be, there's no point in worrying about it.'

Being diagnosed with Parkinson's in their forties didn't stop either Don or Dale from getting on with their lives. Although Parkinson's has changed their lives, as any unpredictable event might, both of them have been positive from the outset about not allowing it to take control. They've utilised whatever support has been available, kept up their fitness through exercise, done everything possible to understand their symptoms, and been open with family and friends about having Parkinson's.

CHAPTER 4

———∞∞∞———

Going Public

When do you tell others you have Parkinson's? Most of us tell family first, usually right after diagnosis, but when to tell friends? This will depend entirely on you, how soon you feel strong enough to say, 'I've got Parkinson's,' and how confident you feel about coping with the inevitable questions.

Telling family and friends

I am very fortunate. I have a husband and two adult children. I have no idea how I would cope on my own. I told them immediately I learned of the diagnosis – my husband first, and then the children. I've never asked them if they suspected anything was wrong, but I don't think they did. My mother was still alive at the time, and she worried when she saw me shaking. I thought I was protecting her by not telling her. Finally, she described my symptoms to her own doctor and asked for an opinion. She then phoned me to report what her doctor had said and told me off for not letting her know myself. I should have told her sooner, but had worried about making her worried, as happens with mothers and daughters.

The main question your children will ask, if they are old enough to consider the implications of the disease, is whether Parkinson's is hereditary. In some cases it is hereditary, but in most it is not. The other reassurance your children need is that they don't have to worry about you; you're still the same person you were before. They get the hang of this after a while, and stop looking at you sideways. But sometimes it's nice to get more hugs and have someone notice when you're fatigued. It also feels good to be complimented on how well you're dealing with Parkinson's.

I'm even more fortunate in having a daughter-in-law, two grandchildren and the prospect of more. The eldest grandchild is still a pre-schooler and has never mentioned my tremor; I do notice other older children watching and I feel self-conscious then. Although none have asked me what the matter is, I wonder when this question will come. I don't want my grandsons to think of me as any different to their other grandmothers (they're lucky enough to have three – one's a step-grandmother). I'm not sure when they might ask me what the matter is, and I'm not sure how I'll respond. It feels a bit serious to say, 'I've got Parkinson's and that makes me shake.' But I prefer this to saying I've got an illness; saying you're ill has all sorts of connotations. Children accept things in a matter-of-fact way and I hope an honest answer will satisfy their curiosity.

One useful and widely available resource for young children is a picture book written by Rasheda Ali, called *I'll Hold Your Hand So You Won't Fall: A Child's Guide to Parkinson's Disease*. Rasheda is the daughter of heavyweight boxer Muhammad Ali, who was diagnosed with Parkinson's in 1984. The book was originally written to help his grandchildren understand why their grandfather couldn't smile.

People from some cultures may prefer to keep the diagnosis to themselves and may refer to it only obliquely. It will help a great deal if the person with Parkinson's can speak openly within the family. There is no need for the diagnosis to go any further than family, medical advisers and caregivers.

Sharing and caring

Many books on Parkinson's have a chapter on the carer or caregiver. The term 'caregiver' is a new one in our lexicon, probably conceived by a social worker reluctant to use the expression 'unpaid servant', though many caregivers now receive payment or a benefit of some kind. Does that still make them givers? If this sounds cynical, it's because the word 'caregiver' scares me so much I didn't want to use it in this book. It means someone who cares for another who can no longer care for themselves. In the case of Parkinson's this is usually a partner.

I don't think of my partner as a caregiver, though he can be very caring. Apart from the fact that I'm no longer working full-time, our life hasn't changed much. I still do all the cooking and most of the cleaning and laundry. This was pretty much the same experience for most women I interviewed; though we might sometimes complain about our partners, we are fortunate in having them to care for us when the going gets tough. I sympathise with those women and men without full-time partners, as they must find it much harder to give up a career which is their primary source of income, and which probably plays a major role in their social life as well; and it must be hard having no one at home to share the tough times.

However, even in such a situation I still think women are more adaptable. They are usually the parent who spends the greater time looking after the children and are more likely to have modified their career to suit family needs. In contrast, a man's career usually takes a predictable path and he is seen most often as the main breadwinner. Should he no longer be able to work, his perceived loss of status can be catastrophic.

Coping with someone who has a chronic illness isn't easy, and even the most caring partner can feel worn out and in need of care themselves. A partner's exhaustion is clearly a signal for time out, no matter what prompts it. If you're the main support person and feel you can't cope any longer, don't be afraid to enlist the help of family or friends.

Once the immediate predicament is over, it might be useful to contact a therapist or other independent and suitably qualified person on whom you can unload from time to time. Apart from private therapy, you may find a local support group for people in a similar situation to yours, or you might look at starting such a group yourself.

We all need support sometimes. The chronic illness of one family member can begin to dominate the life of all within that household. Both the person with Parkinson's and the partner need to be aware of each other's needs and maintain a sense of balance. At different times you will both feel sad, hopeless, frustrated and resentful. You will feel this way simply because you're human.

These feelings may well surface when comforting and loving your partner arouses a desire for greater closeness. Loss of sex drive in a man or woman can cause either them or their partner to feel isolated and rejected. This is usually followed by guilt, which easily turns to anger. You need to talk to each other about your feelings and support each other rather than withdraw. Seek couples guidance counselling if you find it hard to express your feelings without becoming guilty or afraid.

Getting to grips with Parkinson's

When first diagnosed with Parkinson's, you'll want to find out all you can about the disease. You can do most of the initial searching through the internet or local library, but much of what you read is fairly frightening. There's a lot about care and caregivers, special drinking cups and feeding, and walking aids and other things you won't want to think about and don't need to know.

In the beginning I didn't feel the need to talk about Parkinson's with anyone else who had the condition, preferring instead the neutrality of the information on my computer, perhaps because it seemed so remote from me. But there came a time when I wanted to talk to someone else with Parkinson's to find out whether they had the same fear of the future that sometimes overwhelmed me.

I mentioned this to my husband; we could think of two men who had been diagnosed a few years earlier. I was wary in case they might not want to talk about something so personal with a woman. As it happened, they didn't mind; they both helped me by talking about how they'd felt at the beginning (mostly very depressed) and how they were coping now. I was encouraged to hear that apart from adjusted hours, they were both still working. Later, through a friend, I met another man who was also still working, and doing so well that he had even extended his sporting activities to include rowing after being diagnosed eight years earlier. As we all discussed our individual symptoms such as stiffness or tremor, I began to realise that no two people have the disease in the same way. Unlike me, none of them had a tremor, and their other symptoms differed widely.

Buoyed by these meetings, I decided I'd like to meet more people with Parkinson's so I joined the Parkinson's Society. They have a calendar of events and I decided to attend the next meeting. It was not a good experience. Many of those attending were elderly with advanced symptoms, and when I looked at them I slipped back into depression. I felt this wasn't for me and decided not to attend future meetings.

However, I'm fortunate in that I live in the only country in the world where the Parkinson's Society in each region has a trained staff of field officers. These are a trained group of individuals, mostly from medical backgrounds, who work in the field with people like me. They offer advice to clients and their families on everything you want to know about every aspect of Parkinson's. They will probably know more than your medical practitioner because they're working every day with people at all stages. They also assist in accessing services. When you join the society, this free service is yours. Once I had met my particular field officer and learned how she could help me I was hooked, and I really don't know if I would have coped so well without that help.

There are Parkinson's societies in most countries, but few run a system as helpful as this. Most are there to point the patient in the direction of resource material, provide a contact with another person with Parkinson's and a list of support groups run by patients themselves. The UK Parkinson's Society has excellent materials and resources. In the US, neurologists often employ a nurse to work specifically with Parkinson's patients. Although this is better than nothing, it does mean that patients receive only the information that particular neurologist provides; they can get stuck with a single opinion and not have access to neutral advice. My advice to those of you who do not have a field officer service is that you begin to lobby for such a service.

Once I'd joined the Parkinson's Society I could choose what services I required. I learned that one of the field officers was setting up a coffee group for women with early-onset Parkinson's, and this seemed to be just what I had hoped for – a chance to talk with other women closer to my age and with whom I had more in common. The first meeting was held in a café at a local garden centre and was so successful that by the end of it we had agreed on a date for our next meeting.

I've never belonged to sport clubs or joined other social groups, and can appreciate that for some the idea of a support group may be anathema. Being clubbed together with those with whom we have little in common except an illness is not what many of us enjoy. But our group isn't like that. Perhaps meeting in a café helps; I don't think it would work so well if we met in some characterless meeting room. And it doesn't feel like a support group; it seems more like friends meeting over coffee once a month.

You could set up a group like this anywhere in the world, but you will need someone willing to take the responsibility for organising it. Sometimes we might have a guest speaker, or the field officer directs us towards new books, documentaries, research in science and medicine, or services available that might help us deal with Parkinson's more positively. Mostly we share personal experiences and ideas informally. The women's group has proved to be so successful that a men's group has been formed.

Our coffee group is not only a valuable support system; it's a way for those of us of similar age to get together. I'm fairly sure my support group doesn't look like a group of chronic invalids, and none of us would call ourselves elderly, even though Parkinson's is most often associated with the elderly. We like to think we look like any group of women or men meeting for coffee – casual, relaxed and enjoying each other's company.

CHAPTER 5

Secondary Symptoms and How to Manage Them

Finding a combination of any of the primary symptoms of Parkinson's – tremor; bradykinesia or slowing movement; stiffness and rigidity; and loss of balance – will help determine the diagnosis. However, there are also many secondary symptoms. Some are caused by the process of neurological degeneration, and others are a side effect of Parkinson's medication. This chapter covers a broad range of secondary symptoms and offers ways to manage them. The suggestions for dealing with secondary symptoms are drawn from personal experiences. It's a matter of figuring out what works for you.

Depression

Some of you will wonder why you were the one who got Parkinson's, or what you did to cause it, or when might it have begun. Grief, disbelief and depression are natural responses to something so vague in its diagnosis and prognosis; but depression in Parkinson's can also have a physiological cause and even be one of the first symptoms.

I didn't ask myself why I got Parkinson's, but I did feel depressed. It was hard to see the point of a future that offered less quality of life. I discussed these feelings with my neurologist, who suggested I see a neurological psychiatrist. It was good advice; I met someone who understood what I was feeling and why, and prescribed medication to help overcome the depression. I was also relieved to learn that my reaction was fairly normal. Clinically, Parkinson's patients have been found to be significantly more depressed than other chronic illness groups, and depression is thought to be an intrinsic part of the condition; this was recognised as long ago as 1817 when James Parkinson first described the disease.

Technically, the underlying reason for depression is directly related to the loss of dopamine and serotonin in the brain. These 'chemical messengers' or neurotransmitters play a major role in regulating our mood and sense of well-being. They are sometimes described as the 'feel good' chemicals, and people with Parkinson's have reduced levels of both. Consequently, we have more reason than most to feel depressed. Parkinson's has messed with your brain. The electrics no longer flow as freely as they did. Your wiring has been interfered with.

None of this may be overtly obvious – you're not missing an arm or a leg. So how can you say what you've lost? How can you say what your family have lost? If you count the loss of hopes and dreams, that is something to truly grieve over.

I was given a course of serotonin reuptake drugs. Serotonin is one of the neurotransmitters in the brain that allows messages to pass between nerve cells. The theory is that some serotonin is released from the synapse (the space between the cells) during the process of transmission. Selective serotonin reuptake inhibitor drugs (SSRIs) inhibit this process so that the serotonin stays in the synapse longer. This provides greater stimulation of the recipient cell.

SSRIs can be prescribed by a doctor or a psychiatrist, but be aware that some antidepressants are contraindicated with Parkinson's medication. I experienced no problems with the drug I was given, but I've not tried 'coming off' it. Some people experience side effects such as headaches, sweating and nausea while taking or withdrawing from SSRIs.

My own symptoms of depression were mostly a loss of energy and feelings of hopelessness, but symptoms can manifest themselves in many ways. They may include:

+ insomnia
+ loss of energy
+ loss of concentration
+ feelings of hopelessness

✦ poor appetite
✦ irritability
✦ panic attacks
✦ suicidal thoughts.

See your doctor if you have any of these symptoms for more than a week. They may have nothing to do with Parkinson's.

Apathy

Medical professionals now acknowledge that for people with Parkinson's apathy, anxiety or depression can occur quite independently. This means that apathy in a person with Parkinson's should not necessarily be associated with depression but instead be seen as a distinct symptom. My *Roget's Thesaurus* tells me that to be apathetic one 'may be unenthusiastic, unambitious, unimpassioned, uninspired, unexcited, unmoved and incurious'. I know that I can be most unenthusiastic and unexcited at times, but the other descriptions don't seem to apply to me, and no one has suggested I should be screened for apathy. Thinking back, however, to the feeling of hopelessness that I had so long ago, I now wonder whether perhaps that was a sign of Parkinson's apathy. If your doctor is at all concerned, it's important that you are screened so you are not treated for a depressive disorder which you don't have. Should you be diagnosed with apathy your family needs to know that it is a characteristic of Parkinson's; it is not laziness or stubbornness, and cannot be voluntarily controlled.

Currently, there is no medication for neurological type apathy. My only suggestion is physical exercise, brain exercise and company.

Anxiety

Anxiety can be overwhelming. It occurs because the autonomic nervous system sets off false alarms, triggering 'flight or fight' responses. Symptoms may range from mild anxiety to a full-scale panic attack with palpitations, breathlessness, headaches and fatigue. It is no wonder some people become fearful and insecure.

The most commonly reported cause of anxiety is the fear of falling, particularly in public places. This often occurs on stairs, escalators, pavements and discernibly uneven ground.

Sometimes even without realising why, we may become anxious and unable to sleep. One sleepless night may be enough to begin a cycle of anxiety, leading to more sleepless nights; a tremor becomes uncontrollable; muscle tension causes constant pain and more insomnia. Now our symptoms have become much worse and we are truly anxious, fearing that the present has become the future we have been waiting for, the unknown we most fear.

Anxiety can make us feel pessimistic about all kinds of things, big and small. We may need reminding that for every negative thought, there is a positive counter-statement. For example, if you find yourself thinking 'I can't . . .' think 'I can . . .'

If you feel constantly anxious, see your doctor and with their help try to break this cycle. It may require a course of anti-anxiety medication; it may mean a slight alteration to your Parkinson's medication or in some more persistent cases may require cognitive therapy.

Helping yourself get through

Depression, apathy, anxiety – any one of these may cause you to withdraw socially. Doing anything can seem too much of an effort, let alone leaving the security of home to exercise or socialise. I only suggest you try. If your symptoms are seriously disabling, you should seek professional help. Nevertheless, there are some things you can do on your own. Begin by setting some attainable goals, for instance:

- ✦ Get out of bed, shower and have breakfast by 9.00 a.m.
- ✦ Set a timetable for the day.
- ✦ Take a walk with a family member or a friend.
- ✦ Get an exercise programme, join a gym or exercise class.
- ✦ Avoid isolation, unless it's for relaxation.
- ✦ Talk to others who understand your problems.
- ✦ Do something for somebody else.

Show the world a happy face. Even if you have facial masking, don't let it stop you from smiling on the inside.

Stress

Once it was thought stress might be a cause of Parkinson's. We now know this isn't true. However, stress does accentuate the symptoms.

Sources of stress can range from answering the phone or making dinner, to meeting new people, conflicts at work or public speaking.

The stress of coping with your job and Parkinson's can become too hard. Every deadline or disagreement is magnified and symptoms become more pronounced, causing more stress. This is the time when you may have to think of modifying your job or giving it up altogether – a stressful decision in itself and one which also brings grief. Again, remember your family – they will be aware of the pressure you're under, so don't shut them out. Your decision will impact on them as well.

You can try to avoid stress, but a certain amount in life is unavoidable so it's good to learn some tactics for dealing with it, like breathing and relaxation techniques, or joining a yoga laughter group (this is not as silly as it sounds).

Knowing when to ask for help

▶ *Pat was diagnosed with Parkinson's when she was only 50, and that was 14 years ago. Until quite recently she had never experienced stress, in spite of leading a very busy life as a pharmacy assistant and keen sportswoman. She always enjoyed entertaining her friends, till one night she had a meltdown.*

Recently, we asked a couple to dinner, as we were long overdue in issuing a return invitation. When the day came, I had a complete meltdown; I just couldn't go ahead with any preparations. I went to pieces completely, was in tears, shaking like a jelly, and in a real state.

However, I said to myself, 'Come on Pat, you have to solve this.' I phoned my husband at work and he immediately picked up the vibes that I was sending, bless him. So he phoned our guests, made our apologies and dealt with the situation, then came home and calmed me down as well. We took this same couple to dinner at a restaurant at a later date and it all went well.

We need good support around us when we have moments like these, and this was one of those occasions for me.

Fatigue

Parkinson's fatigue can be utterly debilitating – like being empty inside, gutted. It's a tiredness you wake with. You don't want to get out of bed and face the day – you're bone tired, and it's not because you worked yourself to exhaustion the day before. The good news is that it may not be there tomorrow. Don't give in. Be kind to yourself, plod quietly through the day, go to bed early and take your medication on time. Tomorrow you'll probably feel better.

Most of us are tired by mid-afternoon. A rest or a nap helps, along with a boost from an energy drink. Don't take too much sleep during the day, though, or you may find it difficult to sleep at night.

Whatever we do, we need to remember it's going to take longer for us to recover. For example, people with Parkinson's are often surprised that they are exhausted for quite some time after a holiday, even though they coped well and had lots of energy while away.

Disturbed sleep and insomnia

Unfortunately, being tired does not guarantee a good night's sleep. Many of us with Parkinson's develop chronic insomnia. This means that we have an ongoing problem in getting to sleep or staying asleep. Some of us will be woken by vivid dreams and others by rigidity when trying to turn over in bed.

The area in our brain that regulates sleep rhythm is close to the substantia nigra, where loss of dopamine occurs. This could be why people with Parkinson's have sleep problems. But without knowing the definite reason for your sleep difficulties, all you can do is try different ways of easing the problem.

Loss of serotonin (one of the 'feel good' chemicals associated with emotion and mood) causes depression, and this can contribute to sleep difficulties. You won't know if loss of serotonin is the problem until you try an old-fashioned cure to see whether it helps. It's simple: have a drink of warm milk before bedtime. Serotonin is a derivative of tryptophan, which is found in milk. If you don't like warm milk, try hot chocolate or cold milk; warming the milk isn't necessary, it's just for comfort.

I'm fortunate in that mostly I sleep well, and any vivid dreams I have (a possible side effect of levodopa) aren't frightening. A warm bed and warm legs help me relax, but there are bad nights when restless legs keep me awake. The discomfort requires me to walk around the house, waiting for the levodopa to take effect. You may find there are nights when it is useful to have a separate bedroom where you can read, drink your milk or use a relaxation technique until you're able to sleep once more.

I use the following relaxation technique to help me get to sleep, and it works most of the time. It is a variation on meditation or self-hypnosis, and is based on auto-suggestion. Of course it doesn't happen as quickly as it seems here.

Relaxation exercise to encourage sleep

1   Lie on your back.
2   Use a soft pillow and pull the sides around your neck so that your neck and head are supported.
3   Close your eyes.
4   Place your arms on either side of your body. (I usually have to lie on my right hand to stop it shaking.)
5   Try not to think about your tremor. It may take time for it to settle, as it will only happen as you slowly become relaxed.
6   Calm your mind and push away any new ideas that want to intrude. Concentrate only on a point of darkness somewhere ahead. Keep excluding any intrusive thoughts.
7   You will know when you've reached the state of almost sleep, as your tremor will have ceased and you will feel relaxed.
8   Now imagine your mind as an empty circle and you are travelling through the centre of the circle. (This may take time, but be persistent.)

Another way of encouraging good sleep is to ensure you have some light exercise every day. Don't drink caffeine or alcohol or watch a DVD or television just before bedtime, and get to bed around the same time each night. Make your bedtime and waking time habitual by keeping to the same evening routine, if possible. Take your final medication of the day, have a bath or spend a quiet time getting ready for bed, and don't read or watch television in bed.

Some people believe a magnesium supplement helps them sleep by relaxing tight muscles. Others may need professional help; their medication might need altering or it may be suggested that a sleeping pill is tried for a brief period to break the pattern of insomnia. Sleep has to be a habit and is probably the only one we do absolutely need.

Restless legs

The discomfort of restless legs is unusual and truly unpleasant. Restless legs cause a strange sensation which could be described as pain, though it's not an acute pain – it's more like an inner ache. It mostly occurs at night when you've just gone to bed and are trying to get to sleep, but it can also happen when you're relaxing during the day. When it occurs at night, it prompts such a longing to move and relieve your legs of the sensation that sleep is impossible. The condition is not restricted to Parkinson's. Many people suffer from it, but people with Parkinson's seem particularly prone. It may even be an early symptom.

'Restless legs' is a bit of a misnomer, though it does cause an aching inner restlessness when you are trying to get to sleep. Some people describe it as a sensation of something crawling or moving inside the legs. To me it has always felt as if the very essence of the limb is being drawn out through my skin. The compulsion to move relieves the sensation only briefly, and within seconds it returns.

I've found some relief through taking my last levodopa dose of the day about half an hour before bedtime. In this situation you may have to choose between restless legs or the vivid dreams caused by the late-night dose of levodopa. Sometimes I fill a hot water bottle or heat a bean bag and lay this on my knees. The warmth helps to relax the muscles.

Magnesium, calcium and tryptophan supplements have all been suggested to ease this condition. Some studies suggest restless legs could result from an iron deficiency, but don't take iron supplements unless a blood test reveals this is necessary. Instead, make sure you include iron-rich foods such as dark green vegetables, meat and eggs in your diet.

Pain, discomfort, aching

Pain in Parkinson's is difficult to categorise. Many of us experience pain of some kind, ranging from a discomfort, a dull ache or a deep rheumatic-type pain to a sharp radicular pain. It can strike anywhere in the body – the hands, arms, legs, feet and extremities, though usually only one place at a time. For some of us it might be one of the first symptoms.

Pain from a shoulder or the spine can be an early symptom and may be severe enough to require an x-ray, scan or MRI. These are wise precautions, as you may in fact have a trapped nerve or herniated disc. Don't assume the pain is always because of Parkinson's. I took a combination supplement of chondroitin with glucosamine for cartilage development and exercised my way through a frozen shoulder and later a herniated disc. I don't know if there was a connection with Parkinson's or not. Since I was diagnosed I've discovered that many others have experienced back and shoulder pain in the early stages of Parkinson's.

Musculoskeletal pain is a common pain in Parkinson's and is probably related to rigidity and the stiffness of muscles that do not relax properly. This causes muscle cramps and dull aches in arms, legs and joints.

Radicular pain is a sharp shooting pain radiating from pressure or the irritation of a nerve root. It can be part of a tingling or numbness in toes or fingers. It's usually caused by a trapped nerve. I have it as an ongoing problem in my left foot and toes. When an MRI revealed no known problem apart from an unusually high arch, I was advised to use an orthotic sole in my shoe, and this has helped. Otherwise I find massaging my foot seems to restore its equilibrium.

Some of my early experiences with the peculiarity of Parkinson's pain happened long before diagnosis. The first was when my heel became so painful to walk on my doctor suggested I had a heel spur. An x-ray revealed nothing. After some months the pain went away.

I hadn't associated these pains with Parkinson's until I met a number of other people who had experienced almost identical problems. Some said their earliest symptom was a frozen shoulder, others had seen surgeons for a suspected herniated disc and one other had an almost identical problem as mine with his foot.

Parkinson's pain usually occurs when dopamine levels in your system are low, resulting in a greater level of stiffness in joints and muscles. To cope with Parkinson's pain you can take paracetamol (marketed as Panadol or Tylenol) every four hours. If this doesn't help, your doctor may suggest an anti-inflammatory painkiller.

A range of pains

▶ *David is only 49, a keen sportsman who bikes, skis, hikes, boats, swims and maintains a full exercise programme. He was diagnosed with Parkinson's seven years ago.*

David's initial symptom was a frozen shoulder, but then he developed strange pains in his foot. Walking became extremely painful, so much so that he dreaded having to walk anywhere. It felt like a bone spur. Later he developed another pain which felt as if something was stuck in his shoe. This discomfort went on for some time, and then just as mysteriously stopped. Unfortunately, it has recently recurred.

These pains may be described as tingling, numbing, stabbing or sharp, and they are most likely caused by the dysfunctional autonomic nervous system.

David wakes with bad cramps in his right hand at night. His fingers curl up tight and are painful to straighten. His right arm aches and taking levodopa medication hasn't helped much. His job as a technician for nautical instruments such as compasses and sextants requires precision and the ability to deal with fine details. Because of the difficulty of using his right hand, he has taught himself to use his left.

Most days are spent working in his workshop, except when the instruments are fitted into boats when they must be adjusted at sea. He is the only nautical technician in New Zealand and works long hours to keep up with demand from a large boating population.

The eight-hour attention to detail required to complete the delicate work is stressful, and David worries when he gets behind and the work piles up. He knows his work is probably the cause of some of the pain and cramps in his hand and arm, and accepts that he needs to balance work with exercise and relaxation. But he finds it hard to relax when he is worried about his future. He has no idea how long he will be able to handle such fine work. This has been his only career, and he fears the day when he can no longer cope with the precision his job requires.

Some of the painful cramps Dave experiences may be dystonia, a severe spasm or twisting of parts of the body. This can occur in the early morning as a result of lowered dopamine levels. Sometimes it's painless, but at other times it can result in painful cramps as muscles knot into tight contractions and don't relax.

Dystonia

Dystonia is an abnormal cramping muscle spasm or posturing that can occur anywhere in the body, though less often in the hands or arms. It may or may not be painful. Dystonia is most likely a side effect of your medication, and can happen when your drug level is at maximum effect, or when it's low.

Visible signs

▶ *Sometimes dystonia may seem like a permanent feature. That's what worried Kathy most when, not long after she was diagnosed with Parkinson's, she was stricken with dystonia in her face.*

A muscle around my upper mouth was pulling hard on my lip. Dystonia! It embarrassed me and the muscle was beginning to be painful. My children succeeded in making me laugh, by putting a sneer on their faces and giving me examples of sneers that would help me in public. You could say that it was helpful.

The neurologist put me on another medication. It worked brilliantly and both the dyskinesia [involuntary jerky, twisting movements] and dystonia gradually vanished.

My own experience of dystonia has, thank goodness, remained invisible, except when I go barefoot. It's in my toes. I have difficulty finding comfortable shoes as my toes move constantly and rub into blisters and calluses. My right big toe jerks up and down while the smaller toes on both feet curl under.

Some yoga-based exercises are helpful in dealing with dystonia.

Yoga exercise for easing curling toes

This is a calming exercise and will make your feet feel better.

Feet exercise

1   Remove shoes and socks.
2   Stand side on to a wall with your legs slightly apart so you feel well-balanced and grounded. If you wish, you can keep one hand on the wall to steady yourself.
3   Think about how you are standing. Check by looking down the side of each leg to see that your feet are aligned with your hips.
4   Flatten your feet into the ground, taking care not to let them go

over on the side. Don't let the toes curl up or down. You can bend slightly at the knee, if you wish, but don't tighten the buttocks.

5   Imagine your tail bone is pulling down towards the floor.

6   Breathe slowly and consciously. You may hold this position for as long as you like.

Dyskinesia

Dyskinesia is the term applied to abnormal involuntary movements that occur as a secondary problem caused by levodopa. Mostly it is an unpleasant experience, but some people will feel pain before or after an incident of dyskinesia. There's more about dyskinesia in the next chapter on medication and its side effects.

Difficulty walking

One of the characteristics of Parkinson's is a shuffling walk with small steps. It can be seen almost as a tripping forward on the toes. Sometimes when I'm tired, my steps get smaller; I have to pull myself up, think about how I'm walking and stride out. I've also noticed I have a tendency to lean forward, which leads to a hunched look. If you find yourself doing this, place both hands on your hips, a posture that automatically pulls the shoulders back.

An early morning walk will free up your mobility for the day. No matter what the terrain, you need to think about how you walk. If you find yourself starting to take small steps, stride out, lift your toes, put your heels down first, hold your head up and walk tall. Placing heels first also helps prevent falls. If the terrain is rough and you are climbing or stepping over stones, look for hand holds, watch where you're putting your feet, or use a walking stick. Use a handrail going down stairs or an escalator, and don't rush. All my falls have been caused by three things – turning suddenly, rushing, or not lifting my feet.

Nordic walking

Nordic walking has helped many with Parkinson's feel stronger and stride out. It improves posture and balance, strengthens the arms, and loosens the upper body, particularly the chest and shoulders. It challenges the brain to get your body moving in new ways. You do need to be taught by someone trained in Nordic walking to get the maximum benefit.

The walking poles, which are rather like overland ski-poles, are used with alternate arm movements. They provide support and increase confidence, while the rhythm of the fluid upper and lower body movement encourages an evenness of stride. The poles need to fit your height. You can buy poles that concertina for ease of packing into a suitcase or backpack when travelling, but they're not strong enough for continuous use and are more expensive. When done correctly, Nordic walking is an exercise in its own right, but it can also help hikers with Parkinson's keep up with those who walk faster. It can be done alone, with a friend or as part of a walking group.

Micrographia

This literally means 'small writing'. Although it is categorised as a secondary symptom, it's a common symptom of Parkinson's, and sometimes one of the earliest signs of the disease. Our handwriting is so personal. It is our signature, the way we present ourselves to the world, a vanity, a measure of our literary skills. We learn to write at school, and most of us affect a style of handwriting that we think characterises us – neat and tidy, scruffy and careless, intellectual but obscure. So we watch with dismay and bewilderment as our handwriting removes itself from our control and diminishes to resemble an ant's crawl across the page. And it can literally become painful to write.

Luckily, medication usually resolves the problem. My own handwriting is now erratic, untidy, difficult to manoeuvre, sometimes painful to execute, and returns to micro when the effect of the levodopa is low.

Facial masking

Not everyone will experience facial masking, a form of muscle stiffness that results in a flat expression. You may look in the mirror one day and notice you look more severe and find it hard to smile. People with Parkinson's blink less often and our eyes may seem less expressive and slightly staring. Facial masking is more noticeable in those who have had Parkinson's for a long period.

Whenever I notice my expression looks frozen, I try smiling on the inside. I figure that the feeling inside will be conveyed somehow to those around me. I also regularly use facial exercises and massage to keep my muscles toned.

Loss of the sense of smell

Who would have imagined that a movement disorder could diminish your sense of smell? For quite a few people this is an early symptom of Parkinson's. This symptom is not caused by a problem with the autonomic nervous system, but by a lack of dopamine in the olfactory cortex, the part of the brain that receives and processes information about smells inhaled through the nose. Some of us have lost the ability to taste along with the sense of smell. This is because taste is affected by your ability to smell the food you're eating.

Vision problems

For every one of us, regular eye examinations are as important as regular medical and dental check-ups. Regular eye examinations check for major problems, such as glaucoma, cataracts and macular degeneration. But there are particular changes to vision that can arise from Parkinson's. If you have any vision problems, you should see a specialist.

The lack of dopamine can slow the muscle movement of the eyes. This is what reduces the blink rate, which in turn leads to the staring appearance of facial masking, dry eyes and reduced vision. Dry eyes quickly become gritty and tired, making reading difficult. Tear drops or other forms of natural eye wash bought from a pharmacist or optician can relieve this. I've found the simplest and most soothing solution is to bathe my eyes for a few minutes using a hot, wet facecloth as a compress.

Abnormal or limited eye movements make it harder to track objects, judge distances or discern the shape of an object. Our sense of spatial awareness is also altered. I've noticed how often now I misjudge door openings and hit my head or shoulders. I'm no longer so good at estimating spaces when parking my car. I've not experienced any problem with colours, but for some people colours may appear washed out, and clarity is affected.

Usually, levodopa medication eases eye problems and once your neurologist has placed you on this medication you should notice an improvement in your vision, speech and handwriting as well.

CHAPTER 6

Medication Options

At the time of publication there are no medications available to cure Parkinson's. There are medications that can reduce the symptoms and assist in controlling the condition.

The good part is that you may not need to take any medication immediately. This is where my views may differ from others you have read or heard. I see no point in taking any medication until you need it. I began medication later than initially suggested, and when I did, I monitored my reactions carefully in a diary.

When the time comes for you to start taking medication, think carefully. Discuss fully with your neurologist when to take the medication, what to take, and how much. The medications used in treating Parkinson's are not to be taken lightly. What you take in the beginning may determine the future path of the condition.

Obviously, you must rely on the knowledge of your neurologist, but just as important is your ability to understand and communicate your needs. Remember you live with yourself daily, your specialist may see you only once or twice a year. I can't stress enough how important it is that you take some responsibility for your condition. If your neurologist prefers to prescribe and not explain, then emphasise the need for explanation; and if this is not forthcoming, change your neurologist.

When you begin taking medication, try starting off with a low dose. Not everyone needs the same medication or the same amount at the same stage, so it's best not to compare your treatment with that of others. When your neurologist prescribes medication, make sure you understand what type of medication it is, and why he or she thinks it best for you. Write down the pharmaceutical name and the type of medication, and look it up when you get home. If you still don't fully understand, don't hesitate to contact your neurologist, a movement clinic, or your field officer for more information.

There are four main types of medication prescribed for Parkinson's. (I've used the generic names of the drugs throughout, as the pharmaceutical names vary from country to country. Check names in the Glossary.) The main types of medication are: levodopa; dopamine agonists; anticholinergic drugs; and monoamine oxidase B inhibitors.

Levodopa

Levodopa is converted in the substantia nigra to dopamine by dopamine-producing cells, and replaces the natural dopamine lost through Parkinson's. It comes either as a controlled release (CR) drug, which has a hard coating that results in slow absorption, or as an immediate release or regular release drug, which is fast-acting. Controlled release levodopa requires about an hour to take effect and can be taken before or after meal times, but regular release levodopa should be taken 30 minutes before eating, as any food can delay the drug's progress into the small intestine.

Levodopa (marketed as Madopar and Sinemet) is a type of amino acid. Anything that competes with the process of getting it to the brain reduces its effect. Since protein is also high in amino acids, it is the most likely food to impede the progress of the levodopa, so allow an hour between a high-protein meal and your medication.

Getting levodopa to the brain is a complex process. When swallowed with water, the tablet is taken down into the stomach. (See figure on the next page.) From there it is delivered into the small intestine, where the drug is absorbed into the bloodstream by attaching itself to carrier molecules that help it cross the intestinal wall into the blood, and then from the blood into the brain. In the brand of levodopa I take, Sinemet, the drug carbidopa is added to the levodopa to stop it turning into dopamine before reaching the brain.

Levodopa and the digestive system

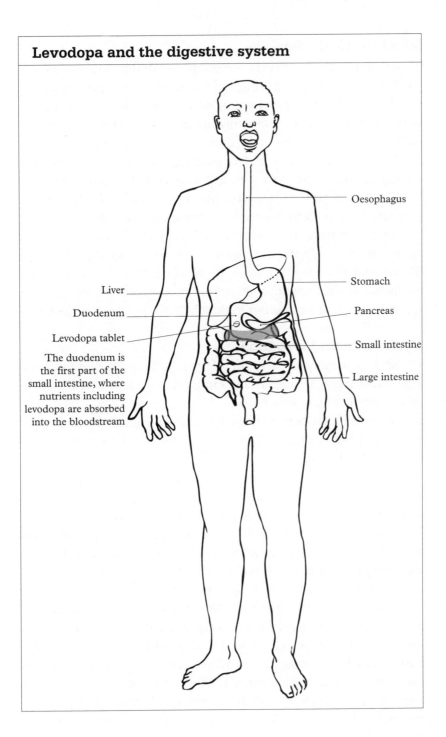

Oesophagus

Liver

Duodenum

Levodopa tablet

The duodenum is
the first part of the
small intestine, where
nutrients including
levodopa are absorbed
into the bloodstream

Stomach

Pancreas

Small intestine

Large intestine

Side effects of levodopa

Three common side effects of levodopa are dyskinesia, nausea and vivid dreams. I began having vivid dreams once I started taking levodopa, and my husband is now used to me talking or calling out in my sleep. Some people have nightmares, but I'm fortunate in that although my dreams are vivid, they are not frightening.

If you develop nausea after your first few doses of levodopa, try taking the medication with a dry cracker. Typically, the body becomes used to the drug and the nausea fades. If the nausea persists, there are anti-nausea tablets you can safely take.

By far the most noticeable side effect of levodopa is dyskinesia, an abnormal involuntary movement that occurs in approximately 40 per cent of people treated with the drug. Dyskinesia manifests as uncontrollable writhing or jerking movements. It seems to be more common in early-onset Parkinson's and results in weight loss.

Dyskinesia and levodopa

Dyskinesia usually occurs when levodopa is at its peak; but the amount, strength, frequency and duration of the levodopa dose may all contribute to this side effect.

When I finally began to use levodopa, I found I couldn't cope with a full tablet of 50/200 controlled release three times a day without developing dyskinesia. I could control the dyskinesia by taking 25/100 CR six times a day in three-hour intervals. This has continued to suit me, and my prescription remains the same today. Whenever I've tried to increase the amount I become dyskinetic. It is now medically accepted that the levodopa dose per kilogram of your body weight is a factor in developing dyskinesia. I weigh only around 45 kg, so it is not surprising that I can cope with less levodopa than someone weighing twice as much as me.

I'm convinced that you learn what dosage suits you best through experience. It's a good idea to keep a record of the time, dose and effect of your levodopa, and to discuss the results with your neurologist before making any adjustments. For me, dyskinesia is the worst side effect of levodopa. It affects my whole body; my entire nervous system feels as though it is being tightened and twisted so much that I can barely think. This, combined with the inability to stop my limbs from jerking, is the most unpleasant sensation I have ever experienced. I prefer the occasional tremor to the discomfort of dyskinesia; in other words I prefer to be slightly underdosed rather than overdosed.

If you develop dyskinesia after taking levodopa, try taking it with a high-protein food, such as a milkshake or a protein drink. The digestion and movement of protein from the stomach to the small intestine hinders the transfer of levodopa into the small intestine and may slow the absorption of the drug.

Levodopa works well in the early stages of Parkinson's because there are still enough dopamine cells in the substantia nigra to convert the drug to dopamine. However, levodopa doesn't prevent the continued loss of dopamine-producing cells. After taking levodopa for a period of time, your response to the drug can start to 'wear off' and become less predictable. Fluctuations may begin to occur between tremor and dyskinesia. This is called 'diphasic dyskinesia', and from this point onwards, finding a balance of medication can be a matter of trial and error. One of the first suggestions your neurologist may make is to modify your medication. In my case, my neurologist has added amantadine (Symmetrel), which is useful in treating restless legs, and ropinirole hydroxide (Ropinirole, Requip), a dopamine agonist which already has decreased the dyskinesia.

Dopamine agonists

Dopamine agonists stimulate some of your dopamine receptors without needing to change into dopamine. They are not as effective as levodopa. They may be used early in Parkinson's and delay the need for levodopa, or they may be prescribed at a later stage along with levodopa to extend its effectiveness and smooth out problems of a sudden drop-off in the level of effective levodopa. They are particularly useful if you have dyskinesia.

They may have relatively ordinary side effects, such as dizziness, drowsiness and nausea. However, some people may develop bizarre behaviours known as impulse control disorders. These include pathological gambling, excessive shopping, eating or heightened sexuality. These impulses are often embarrassing and shameful, and people may not associate them with their medications and may be reluctant to tell anyone or seek help. Sometimes the disorder develops after an increase in medication, and high doses of agonists do seem to increase the risk.

Your neurologist should inform you of these potential problems and discuss them fully before prescribing, and if you think you have developed a problem you should let your doctor know immediately. Something as simple as decreasing the dose slightly may help. But don't exclude dopamine agonists as a medication option; they provide great benefit to most of us prescribed them. They've helped stop the dyskinesia I was so troubled with and I wouldn't want to give them up. Incidentally, I wonder how many of us with Parkinson's have always tended towards being obsessively perfectionist. Is there such a thing as a Parkinson's personality?

Anticholinergic drugs

Anticholinergic drugs were used to treat Parkinson's before the development of levodopa. They apply the brakes on your tremor by blocking the action of acetylcholine, one of the neurotransmitters. When dopamine is low, acetylcholine can prompt an excess of stimulation, causing tremor and rigidity. Anticholinergics may block this effect. Like most Parkinson's drugs, they are not without possible side effects, such as dry mouth, constipation and hallucinations.

Amantadine

This drug is also called Symmetrel. It was not developed as a Parkinson's drug and differs in this way from the others mentioned. Amantadine was originally developed to prevent and treat influenza. One day in 1967 a Parkinson's patient who had taken amantadine to overcome flu symptoms discovered her Parkinson's also improved. Tests made at the time showed that amantadine did increase dopamine perhaps by blocking the neurotransmitter acetylcholine. I took this drug prior to beginning levodopa, and am trying it again to treat diphasic (wearing off) dyskinesia. The side effects of amantadine can be swollen or discoloured legs.

Contraindications of other drugs

Taking medication for Parkinson's can cause complications with other drug treatments. This could happen, for example, if you took ill while travelling or had to see a doctor unfamiliar with your condition. Some people choose to wear a medical-alert bracelet to notify their condition to anyone attending them, if they become unconscious or are unable to speak for themselves. Whenever you see a new doctor, dentist or other health professional who may need to prescribe medication, you need to tell them what Parkinson's medications you are taking so they can check for any contraindications. There are booklets on the drug treatment of Parkinson's that inform you of any contraindications with other drugs. Most Parkinson's websites in each country will provide this information. If you don't have access to such information, make sure your doctor or dentist checks for you.

Those medications that may require caution include:

+ anaesthetics prior to surgery
+ antidepressants (certain types only)
+ anti-emetics
+ antihistamines
+ cardiovascular medication
+ cold and cough medicines
+ enlarged prostate medication.

Coping with medication

Once you begin medication it's important to take it properly. Like much of everything else about coping with Parkinson's, you need to be responsible. Establish a timetable for your dosage and stick to it. Follow the same routine each day. If you're travelling, leave your watch on home time until you're settled.

Measure your tablets out each morning and place the day's dose in a separate pillbox (some pharmacists will do this for an extra charge). I've found this is the only way I have of checking that I've taken all my tablets and at the correct time. Take the pillbox with you wherever you go. It's always useful to have a spare pill container in your bag as well, particularly for those times when you rush out without thinking and realise you've left your medication at home. If you miss a dose and remember a bit later, take it then and keep to the time for the next one. If you don't remember until the time of the next dose, don't take two to make up for the one you missed. And don't stop taking your medication unless your neurologist advises you to do so.

Taking tablets at regular intervals outside the usual breakfast, lunch and dinner times can be hard to remember. Some people use an alarm clock, either on their mobile phone or on a special pill container (though this can attract unnecessary attention when the alarm goes off). I prefer to take medication as surreptitiously as possible.

You will probably need to adjust your medication from time to time, and there may then be a period of adjustment to a new medication. Should you develop bothersome side effects during this time let your neurologist know. Fine-tuning can sometimes be complex. Getting a balance between too much or too little of any drug should be a process shared between you and your doctor. It's a good idea to monitor your response, whether for better or worse, and always keep your neurologist informed. Don't wait for your next appointment.

Getting the balance right

▶ *Robyn was diagnosed four years ago, and she's now 57. She's a keen golfer, like her husband. Robyn says they spend most of their leisure time on golf courses and even their holidays become golfing holidays. Her life with Parkinson's was going reasonably smoothly until she developed dyskinesia.*

Robyn says the dyskinesia happened quite suddenly. Her medication was no longer helping her and instead had begun hindering her ability to do all her usual activities. Because of dyskinesia, she rapidly lost weight and found it difficult to still her twisting frame. She tried various suggestions from friends, such as having a milkshake or protein snack at the time of taking her levodopa tablets, but none of these helped. She waited until the next appointment with her neurologist, by which time she had lost considerable weight. He suggested adding another medication, amantadine, to her treatment, and since then she has returned to her usual self, except none of her clothes fit and she's had to use food supplements to help put some of the weight back on.

For someone as proud of her fitness as she was, it was tough when her medication let her down, but now with the balance provided by the amantadine she's back to being always on the go, either working, exercising, playing golf or picking up various grandchildren from pre-school. She has two children of her own and four stepchildren, along with six grandchildren, so family life is busy. She also works with her husband in his business.

She still has a tremor sometimes in her hand and left leg, and occasional numbness in her left foot. When she's overtired she's 'all over the place' and says it's hard to keep still. Sleep is probably now her biggest problem. She goes to sleep easily, but wakes after about an hour, then seems to stay awake for hours.

Her experience with dyskinesia has made her more concerned about the long-term future, mostly about losing her independence, being obviously different to the capable woman she is now, becoming a burden on her family and not being able to play golf with her husband and friends. She says it's silly, but one of her big worries is that she'll end up wearing a tracksuit and trainers and accidentally knocking goods off the shelves in the supermarket when her arm swings wildly.

Levodopa has given those of us with Parkinson's the opportunity of a close to normal life. When levodopa seems to lose its effectiveness, it's easy to feel that maybe this is the end of that cosy friendship; we naturally become despondent. Yet, as we know, there are other drugs, such as the anticholinergics, the agonists and amantadine, that can improve our response to levodopa and get us moving again. So if this happens to you, do see your neurologist. Be prepared for a little trial and perhaps some error, and get your medication working for you again.

CHAPTER 7

New Treatments

S omeone will always be telling you about the latest developments
for a cure for Parkinson's – they might have read about a new
drug or surgical procedure, or seen a documentary on television
about stem cells. In reality, a great deal of research is being done,
but we're still mostly relying on the discovery of levodopa more
than 40 years ago for treating Parkinson's. If you wish to know more
about any of the treatments discussed here, I suggest you ask your
neurologist.

Pharmaceutical research

There is a great lack of public understanding of what's involved in
trialling a new medication. The research has to be thorough, so it
takes about 15 years to get a new product ready for the market –
that is, if it doesn't fail somewhere along the way. So far nothing
comparable to levodopa has been found. However, pharmacological
research is ongoing, and along with it the hope of finding a miracle
drug.

The closest success was observed by chance in the dubious
form of the narcotic ecstasy; the case featured in a BBC *Horizon*
documentary called 'Ecstasy and Agony'. A young man who had
been diagnosed with Parkinson's five years previously and had
developed severe dyskinesia took the illicit drug ecstasy one night
while out clubbing. His body was suddenly free of Parkinson's
symptoms and levodopa side effects; he could move freely while the
effect of the ecstasy lasted.

He later underwent a series of observational medical tests in the hope that one day the findings would lead to a new Parkinson's drug. He was variously given levodopa, ecstasy and a placebo. Surprisingly, a brain scan showed that the ecstasy triggered the neurotransmitter serotonin and not dopamine. Yet for some unknown reason, the effect on his Parkinson's symptoms matched that of the dopamine response he received from his initial doses of levodopa. Anyone with Parkinson's is strongly advised against using this recreational drug. Ecstasy is known to be toxic to remaining dopamine-producing neurons. The consequences of taking this drug could be a permanent worsening of the Parkinson's and possibly result in other brain damage.

Currently, once you develop complications such as dyskinesia, successful medication becomes difficult. Keep a diary of how your body is reacting, so that your neurologist has a better chance of working out what is going on. This makes it easier for them to successfully manipulate your medication in various ways. There is another option that may be offered to you at this time, and that is surgery.

Surgical procedures

There are several surgical procedures offered for the treatment of Parkinson's. The operations you might have heard of are pallidotomy (an early procedure to cauterise an area of the globus pallidus, now very rarely used); thalamotomy (which focuses on a part of the brain called the thalamus); and deep brain stimulation (DBS).

Pallidotomy and thalamotomy were the earliest surgeries, both involving cauterisation, and both mostly now replaced by DBS. Thalamotomy seemed to help people with few symptoms other than a serious tremor. The procedure focuses on the thalamus, which receives and relays input from all parts of the brain to the primary sensory areas of the cerebral cortex. During the procedure the patient remains awake, and anaesthesia is applied locally. The area of the thalamus to be treated is identified by a CT or MRI scan, and a needle is inserted to cauterise the overactive part that's causing the aberrant electrical activity. The cauterisation impedes the flow of overactive impulses; it also destroys a small part of the thalamus. Although the symptom of tremor may subside immediately, it can reappear as the area heals. As this procedure involves the destruction of part of the thalamus, it has now been largely replaced by DBS, which does not cause permanent damage.

Deep brain stimulation (DBS)

DBS is a surgical procedure begun in a similar manner to a thalamotomy. The area of the brain usually targeted is the subthalamic nucleus, which is close to the dopamine-producing substantia nigra, and was previously thought to have no connection to Parkinson's, as it didn't produce dopamine. However, studies of the subthalamic nucleus found it was hyperactive in people with Parkinson's (Luo et al., 2002). The neurotransmitter in the subthalamic nucleus was identified as glutamate; it was hoped this would lead to the development of a pharmacological drug for Parkinson's. So far this hasn't happened. Instead, it was found that DBS on the subthalamic nucleus or the globus pallidus interna relieves Parkinson's symptoms (Follet et al., 2010).

During the procedure an electrode is implanted in the chosen implant area so that an electric current can be used to stimulate the aberrant area. The shocks seem to jolt the area back into normal activity. Two operations are required: one to place two wires with electrodes permanently into the targeted region; another to implant wires from the electrodes to a small computer beneath the skin under the collarbone, rather like a heart pacemaker. Electricity flows from this device through the electrodes into the brain and returns to the computer to close the circuit. The batteries in the computer device will last for three to five years before needing to be surgically replaced.

The success of DBS depends on teamwork, time and preparation by the neuropsychiatrist, neurosurgeon, anaesthetist and an ongoing support group. Patients have to be carefully assessed for their suitability to undergo the operation and their chances of success. DBS only improves motor function, so if there are other, more problematic symptoms, they will remain and may become more noticeable later. Like any operation, DBS is not without risks, particularly those associated with any major surgery, such as infection, bleeding and device-related complications. The procedure is not a cure, but for some who have developed dyskinesia to a point where they can no longer function, it can provide immediate relief and make it possible to live a much fuller life.

Deep Brain Stimulation (DBS)

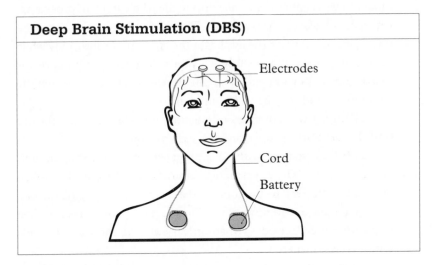

Undergoing DBS

▶ *Les realises now that he would have only been about 26 when he developed the first signs of Parkinson's. He didn't realise what it was at the time and continued his studies. After graduating with a PhD in chemistry, he was looking forward to the career that normally follows years of study. Then his health began to deteriorate and at the age of 34 he was diagnosed with Parkinson's.*

Over the next ten years there was a steady decline in his ability to work, and he relied more and more on his parents and his partner. His main problem became achieving a balance between the medication and dyskinesia.

Finally, his neurologist suggested that it might be possible to overcome the dyskinesia using DBS in the subthalamic nucleus. He referred Les to another neurologist for a second opinion and then to a movement clinic where Les and his partner met the movement disorder nurse. After a number of psychological and neurological tests, Les was scheduled for surgery at a hospital some distance from his home town. What follows is Les's diary of the events from the time he and his partner met the neurological surgeon. (Prior to acceptance into the DBS programme a patient undergoes tests including psychological and psychiatric assessments.)

19 July: Our introduction to the neurological surgeon consisted of a brief run-through of operational procedure, our expectations, etc. I was very apprehensive before this consultation. Up to this point I thought I was going to be awake during the whole implant procedure, which could take up to eight hours. Thankfully, the surgeon corrected this – I was not going to be awake for the entire procedure, only while they were placing the electrodes. After this meeting my mind was eased, knowing I had made the right choice of surgeon, and that the operation would only be 2–8 hours long.

23 July: I was admitted to hospital, introduced to the theatre staff. Lovely warm people, and felt very welcome.

24 July: I woke up with no apprehensions, no expectations and no medications. The anaesthetist reminded me I would be woken during the surgery to do some tests. They shaved my head. The operation took just over two hours. During the operation I was woken to position the electrodes; I had an eerie feeling for a few seconds until I realised where I was.

While awake, I felt no pain. They positioned the electrode and asked me to wiggle my hand, then repositioned it and so on. Once they were satisfied the two electrodes were in the correct place they put me back to sleep. When I woke, my main concern was about the medications I had with me and what I would be given by the hospital. I had put my tablets in a single container, and although I knew what was what, the hospital weren't keen to allow me to self-medicate.

25 July: I'm still on my usual medications. Received an early visit from the surgeon, who was excited at how well the operation had gone and by my own progress. He was ready to proceed to the next stage, normally done a week later.

26 July: I'm still on my usual medications. Early evening went into theatre for Stage 2 of the DBS procedure. This is when they implant control units and battery packs, then wire them up to the electrodes. The wires are placed under the skin behind the ears and down and around the back of the neck, then across the chest to the control unit. It's a 3–4-hour operation, and there were no problems.

27 July: This is the big day. The surgeon arrived at the crack of dawn and turned on the electrodes that were to last me for the next five years. I had weird feelings like pins and needles at first, but they disappeared quickly. The moment the power was turned on I was reborn. The effect of DBS was instant. I could move, walk, talk and function better immediately. At the same time my medication was reduced dramatically.

28 July: My progress is exceptional. I've recovered rapidly, much to the amazement of the surgical team. Feel like I've swallowed an Energiser battery. I was allowed out of the hospital for lunch and nothing could stop me. I wanted to walk everywhere and eat everything. I've not been able to eat a decent meal for ten years. I felt as alive as I had felt 20 years ago.

30 July: My quality of life has undergone an exceptional improvement. I'm still recovering and getting used to seeing the wires just under the skin in my chest. They look a bit like a vein and take a little bit of getting used to when I turn my head. I was discharged from hospital and moved to a nearby hotel for a 3–4-week recovery period. During that time I received follow-up sessions every 3–4 days for adjustments to the control panels before returning home.

One year later, 23 July: My medication is down to only 2½ tablets of levodopa a day. My quality of life is excellent. Sometimes I have a slight speech impediment when my medication is wearing off.

DBS has improved my day-to-day life beyond my wildest dreams. I don't have to wake up every 2–3 hours through the night to take medication. The apparent carpal tunnel syndrome in my right hand has disappeared. I am able to swallow properly, I can sleep for 6–8 hours through the night, and I don't freeze any more. My bladder control has improved dramatically.

I am grateful to the medical, surgical and nursing staff involved, particularly the movement clinic nurse, who although not present, kept in contact during the recovery period and provides ongoing support.

Stem cell transplantation

One of the most talked about new procedures for neurological disorders such as Parkinson's is stem cell transplantation. Developments in the use of stem cell transplants in Parkinson's appears to be full of promise, but there are some big hurdles to overcome before we reach the stage of practical application.

What are stem cells?

We all begin life as a single cell, a fertilised egg called a blastocyte. This single cell cleaves into two cells and in the first five days rapidly multiplies into a multi-cell organism. The inner cell mass of the blastocyte contains stem cells, known as embryonic stem cells. These have the ability to turn into more than 200 different kinds of cells in our body – heart cells, skin cells, neural cells.

Transplantation of embryonic stem cells

The major source of embryonic stem cells suitable for use in transplants has been in-vitro fertilisation (IVF), when the number of eggs fertilised is more than is needed to be implanted in the uterus. It is the process of IVF that has offered scientists a much greater understanding of stem cells.

Embryonic stem cells are the uncommitted cells taken from a blastocyte (fertilised egg) in its first three to five days of existence. They can be directed to become any cell type in the body, undergo 'self-renewal' and make copies of themselves. This means scientists can take a few stem cells and expand the number in a culture dish indefinitely. Stem cells can then be directed to become immature brain cells (neural precursor cells) by applying chemicals while growing the stem cells in a culture dish.

All this is currently possible. However, once the stem cells have been turned into immature neural precursor cells, they need to be transplanted into the brain before they mature, otherwise they will not be able to integrate and make connections within the neural pathways. In the case of Parkinson's, they ideally need to be implanted directly into the basal ganglia where they can begin to produce dopamine directly.

It sounds simple, but there are problems. The biggest one is that some uncommitted embryonic stem cells may be transplanted into the brain along with the neural precursor cells. Unfortunately, the transplant has to be done before it's possible to know whether uncommitted cells are present, and these uncommitted stem cells could develop into tumours. Other issues that need to be resolved by scientists include how to ensure the transplanted neural precursor cells form the right type of connections and behave in the manner of mature brain cells.

There are also problems to do with tissue rejection after transplantation due to immunological incompatibility between the patient and the donated embryonic stem cells. The ideal source of stem cells for transplantation therapy may therefore be adult stem cells which are obtained directly from the patient.

Adult stem cells

In our adult brain, as in some other parts of our body, there are uncommitted stem cells with the potential to become specific mature cells or tissue. The problem is how to get them to where they are needed. The biggest source of neural stem cells is locked away in a part of the brain far from the substantia nigra and there seems no way of accessing them without opening up the space containing them. Unfortunately, this space is also the source of spinal fluid. Scientists have observed adult stem cells travelling from this space into the Parkinson's-diseased basal ganglia, almost as if the brain is trying to heal itself. However, for some reason once these stem cells have reached the area very few of them survive, so sourcing adult stem cells from the Parkinson's-affected brain, directing them to differentiate and implanting them back into the basal ganglia seems problematic. Trying to understand how to enhance the self-repair process may offer a strategy that uses the patient's own stem cells without a need for transplantation. Adult stem cells from other regions such as the umbilical cord, blood or bone marrow may also provide another source by which to obtain stem cells for transplantation. Stem cells from these sources have been shown to have a protective and anti-inflammatory effect in brain injury and disease.

Induced pluripotent stem cells

Induced pluripotent stem cells are generated from skin cells obtained from a skin biopsy (pluripotent means they have the potential to become any type of cell). Adult skin tissue cells can be taken from a patient and genetically 'reprogrammed' to regress and become just like embryonic stem cells. As with embryonic stem cells, these cells can be grown in culture dishes and then directed to become neural precursor cells. While this technology offers the ability to use cells obtained directly from the patient, thus removing issues of tissue rejection, the same issues of tumour formation exist.

I would suggest that you strongly question any miracle stem cell claims made to you by seeking advice from your neurologist or from your local Parkinson's Society.

Gene therapy

Gene therapy is another new treatment being tested for use in illnesses like Parkinson's that are currently incurable. It is hoped that gene therapy will offer an alternative for people with Parkinson's for whom surgery is not an option and who have developed side effects from the drugs they are taking. The technique involves inserting a healthy copy of a gene into the damaged area.

Each cell in your body (except for red blood cells) has an entire copy of your DNA blueprint. A small segment of DNA that codes for a protein is called a gene. Our genes are like barcodes on items in a supermarket. They carry the specific instruction code for the many different proteins that are found in our cells, so that different cells produce different selections of proteins – that's why a brain cell is different to a kidney cell. Gene therapy basically involves using synthetic copies of a gene (or other forms of genetic material) to target the instruction blueprint encoded in our DNA and alter the way a cell normally behaves. Essentially, the overall goal of introducing a synthetic gene is to provide some therapeutic benefit.

In Parkinson's, the cells that produce dopamine are progressively dying. An example of a gene therapy strategy might be to introduce a synthetic copy of a gene that codes for a protein capable of boosting the resistance of cells that are destined to die, or protects them from whatever it is that is attacking them. To prevent the body rejecting these introduced genes, they are delivered via vehicles called 'vectors' derived from harmless non-pathogenic viruses. Once they have delivered the cargo safely to its destination, the viruses are deactivated.

One type of virus used for gene therapy is known as an adeno-associated virus (AAV). Although a large proportion of the human population has been exposed to AAV, it has never been associated with human disease. In gene therapy, the virus is modified to encase a synthetic copy of the targeted gene. Imagine AAV is like a chocolate with a filling in the centre. The shell of a chocolate is the AAV part that helps deliver the filling (the synthetic gene) inside it. We can change the filling to whatever synthetic gene we need, but the AAV shell remains constant. The strategy of gene therapy is that once AAV gets into a cell, it will safely deliver the synthetic gene.

This technique was trialled in a small group of people with Parkinson's. Called a Phase 1 trial, its primary goal was to show the safety of the procedure and how the patients coped, and whether they had unexpected side effects or became ill (Kaplitt *et al.*, 2007). The AAV used in the trial carried a synthetic copy of a gene called glutamic acid decarboxylase (GAD), which is an enzyme involved in producing GABA, a neurotransmitter that is the main inhibitor in the brain. It calms the cells in the subthalamic nucleus that have become over-excited from being deprived of dopamine.

The type of AAV used preferentially targets neurons. This is because neurons have proteins on their outer surface called receptors that AAV binds to. Put simply, you could visualise it as an AAV vector having a 'key' (in facts lots of them) on their outer surface and the neurons having the correct 'lock' on their outer surface allowing them to engage with each other and ensuring successful implantation of the GAD gene.

The criteria for enrolment in the trial and the surgical procedure itself were similar to those used in deep brain stimulation or DBS. Patients needed to be awake and so received only a local anaesthetic in the scalp. The surgeon inserted a probe that measured electrical activity as it passed through the brain to the subthalamic nucleus, which has a distinct electrical signature. On reaching the target site a thin catheter was inserted through the hollow centre of the probe and a few droplets of the AAV infused into the subthalamic nucleus. The probe was removed, the scalp sewn and the patient transferred to intensive care for monitoring.

In a Phase 1 trial, the primary goal is to demonstrate the safety of the procedure. Looking at whether it produces an improvement is not one of the primary goals; but if there is an improvement, that is a bonus. In the first trial, the results showed that the procedure was safely tolerated by the patients, they had no adverse side effects associated with the gene therapy, the gene therapy didn't make the Parkinson's symptoms worse, and some of the patients actually showed a 27 per cent improvement in motor function on the side that received the treatment. The success of that trial led to a second gene therapy trial, a Phase 2 trial aimed at looking at whether the gene therapy could improve movement in a separate group of patients. The results of this Phase 2 trial showed patients receiving genuine gene therapy had an average 23 per cent improvement in motor functions, compared with 13 per cent for those who received sham surgery (Lewitt *et al.*, 2011). A Phase 3 trial is now being planned.

Research into new ways of administering levodopa

Because levodopa loses some of its effectiveness when administered orally, new ways of administering it into the stomach are being explored. Subcutaneous apomorphine is a dopamine agonist that can be injected by the patient through a tube fitted into the stomach. Duadopa is a gel containing levodopa and carbidopa that is administered automatically into the duodenum by an external programmed pump. Both procedures require surgery under a general anaesthetic to insert the tube. Because of the potential for complications, neither procedure is readily available.

——— ⦿ ———

CHAPTER 8

Employment and Work

When you receive a diagnosis that turns your life from known to unknown, it's very hard to go to work the next day as if nothing has happened. Yet that is what most of us have done. While your body may not be functioning quite as well as it used to, in many ways nothing has changed because of the diagnosis – you're still the same person you were yesterday and you'll still be the same person next week.

Your symptoms may take years to progress to a point where they cause you major difficulties. Should you resign today because in eight years you might not be able to do the job? Of course not! You don't need to make any major decisions now.

Gradual changes

▶ *About seven years before I was diagnosed, I remember standing in the shower one morning and feeling an overwhelming sense of hopelessness. I had been self-employed for years as a producer of documentaries and theatre. I loved doing what I was doing.*

I've no idea what happened or why it was that day, but the loss of hope was so all-pervading, I knew the drive to succeed as an independent producer had gone and I didn't even care. I didn't work competitively again. Instead, I started working for other producers as a researcher, a job I thoroughly enjoyed and was still doing when diagnosed.

I'm confident now that what I felt that day was an early indication of Parkinson's. Feelings such as hopelessness are often associated symptoms because of the loss of the 'feel-good' chemical dopamine in the brain. What I felt was not associated with any external factors, and was so extreme that it had to have some other cause. I have experienced it again since diagnosis, but never as powerfully as on that day.

Finally, it was the stress of working in television that got to me. I became worried and anxious about things that I would normally have coped with. I couldn't deal with arguments, and opinionated people love arguing. I was overly anxious about finance and the process of applying for funds. I could no longer cope with conflict or rejection. When I became stressed, my tremor got worse. I was embarrassed when this happened in meetings, especially when most of the others in the room were younger. I imagined they were thinking 'She's losing it!' I remember one day, some time before my diagnosis, I was walking upstairs with some actors. My arms were filled with documents and I lost my balance and fell. I was overwhelmed by embarrassment, and my confidence plunged with me. Whatever anyone else thought, I have no idea and I've never asked. As soon as I finished that project, I gave away television for good.

After I was diagnosed, I started working for a friend who was setting up a fashion business. The hours were good and it was great having no responsibility except for selling beautiful clothes, which I loved wearing as well. At the end of the day I could go home and not think about work until the next day.

For a couple of years things went well. Then the tremor started getting worse. I would be fine until someone asked to try something on or needed advice. I was sure they must think I was shaking because I was inadequate, not telling the truth, or worse still, that I had a drinking problem. I'd tell them it was Parkinson's and then they'd feel sorry for me, and soon it was all too much for me. I had to leave.

We'd just bought an apartment, and it felt like time for a complete change. I'd also been doing volunteer work with an organisation helping victims of domestic violence. I left them too. I felt I needed time just for me, and to sort out our new environment. Life changes all the time. There's always something new to do, and sometimes you get paid for it and sometimes you don't.

Having confessed how it was for me, it may seem strange that I now suggest you should try not to dwell on how Parkinson's might affect your work until it does. My experience is just an example, and it took place over a number of years. Don't leap into thinking your career is over as soon as you've been diagnosed. Evaluate your circumstances by all means, but don't rush to sudden conclusions or make rash decisions.

In certain jobs you will need to let your employer know about your condition as soon as possible, either for health and safety reasons, or because your employment contract requires you to disclose any illness. In either case, it is best to tell your employer as early on as possible; they may be more sympathetic.

Keep in mind that whenever you choose to discuss your health with your employer, it could prompt a re-evaluation of aspects of your job. Even after you have accepted that you need to adjust your workload, you may be unprepared for your change of status in the workplace. The resulting loss of social standing can be quite overwhelming and may lead to a diminished sense of self-worth.

Remember that Parkinson's should not define you in your workplace, or anywhere. You are the same person with the same skills and knowledge as before – you just happen to have Parkinson's. Most of us who've had Parkinson's for some years now have been able to adapt working life to suit – perhaps not always as we'd hoped, but then life wasn't meant to be simple.

Changing roles at work

▶ *Although Michael is 66 and of retiring age, he feels that Parkinson's has forced him to take early retirement from a successful career in management. He now works as a part-time sales person for the company he once managed. Michael has shown dignity in accepting a lesser role.*

The big challenge for me has been to deal with my career. As my symptoms became more obvious, I knew I would have to come to terms with standing down from the position of managing a large department store, a job which carried considerable status.

I had discussions with directors of the company board, explained my situation and what I felt I could offer the company from now on. I never considered leaving the company altogether and I never said a word to my staff. I continued doing my work and carrying this emotional baggage with me until the time finally came when I had to inform loyal staff of my change in status, and why. What followed was an emotional meeting with lots of tears, and for me a terrible sense of wondering what the change would mean in reality.

I have had over 20 years in Toastmasters International, during which time I have listened to some wonderful speakers. I remember one particular speech entitled 'The Art of Leadership'. I took from this a statement that said when your term of leadership ends, walk away, and do not turn around and look back. This became my mantra and I believe it has helped me get through the change in my career.

I have had no desire to stop working and hope to keep doing so for as long as possible, but I have had to accept a complete change of status. After being a manager for most of my working life I decided to stay with the company in the position of salesman.

Initially, this was very hard. I had to take instruction instead of giving it, and I suffered a loss of dignity and standing, but the goal posts had shifted and the best thing I could do was to get on with life. After some time I decided it wasn't too bad after all. I had a job; the wage was certainly not what I'd been used to, but the people I worked with respected me and seemed to enjoy my company.

So how does the future look now? I have the love and support of my family; I am respected at work; and my lifelong friends are there for me. I still have my down days when the body won't do what I want it to (and this is something I am learning to live with). I am sometimes quite emotional, and can become a little depressed when I see some of my new Parkinson's friends deteriorate, and I wonder if I will be like that.

I find comfort and solace in going to the synagogue on Saturday mornings where I can seek some divine help from a higher power. My elder twin brother died suddenly a year ago, which was very sad, but I take these knocks in my stride because there is nothing I can do to bring him back. I know that Parkinson's will not kill me, that I will die with it not of it, so I do the best I can with each day in the knowledge that there will be a cure out there some time.

I remember when my father died suddenly at the age of 52, my mother called us together. She opened a diary and turned the pages over to a new page and said, 'This is the end of the story with father in our lives. Now we must move on and begin a new chapter, because nothing can change it back to what life was like with father.' With these thoughts in my head I have moved on and accepted that this is the way life is for me now.

Michael has accepted a huge change in status and salary, for which he is to be much admired, but for which he was quite unprepared.

Working with your employer

Parkinson's is unusual. There are not many degenerative diseases that you live with for a long time, but don't die from. It could be many years before you reach retirement age. So at what point are you unable to work to the best of your ability, and when is it reasonable to expect an employer to modify the work environment to cope with your Parkinson's?

In most Western countries the Human Rights Act makes it unlawful for an employer to discriminate against anyone with a disability, and requires that when necessary the workplace and/or conditions of employment should be modified to allow the employee to remain in the job. There are two exceptions to this general rule – when the modifications required are unreasonable (not just in terms of cost), or when keeping the disabled employee employed threatens the safety of other workers.

You may decide not to disclose you have Parkinson's until your symptoms make it necessary. However, it is important that you check any legal obligations to disclose your disease at the time of diagnosis – for example, your employment contract may contain a clause that requires disclosure, particularly if there's a risk that not doing so could put you or others in danger in your workplace. If you have any doubts, consider getting legal advice.

Your employer cannot change your contract without your agreement, unless it is clearly stipulated in the contract that they can do so – such as amending normal hours of work because of business needs. You have a right to have a support person at any meeting with your employer to discuss your future with the organisation. It is a good idea to prepare an agenda before any such meeting so that you feel in control and don't forget anything.

Ensure your employer understands Parkinson's disease; have some information available. If you're required to be assessed by an independent medical practitioner (occupational physician), make sure you see one who understands Parkinson's, or request one who does. Record any agreed variations of your employment contract in writing, and get legal advice if you need it.

If you are unfairly dismissed because of your illness, you can challenge the dismissal by raising a personal grievance, or a complaint of unlawful discrimination; there may be a time frame within which the notification should be made. Policy differs from one country to another, but in many countries you can't pursue a complaint under the Human Rights Act as well as a personal grievance under the Employment Relations Authority; you can, however, use the mediation services provided by both agencies without compromising your choice of either, and both are available if the grounds of grievance differ.

Remember your skills and experience are of value to your employer. They may be happy to modify your workplace and employment contract. Whatever approach you take will depend on your individual circumstances and would be best decided after discussion with your lawyer.

Other matters to consider

By definition, every person with early-onset Parkinson's will be of working age, yet only a small number will be insured against loss of income. Some might have partners capable and willing to support them. But what do the others do?

If you are a member of a group health policy, sick leave policy or group income protection policy, seek advice on the insurance benefits you're entitled to. A group policy should be able to be transferred to an individual policy without loss of entitlements or allowances for pre-existing conditions. If you experience problems, seek legal advice.

The value of legal advice

▶ *Clare is in her mid-fifties, and divorced with two adult children. She was formerly a chartered accountant and effectively retired two years ago.*

As an accountant, my immediate thought upon diagnosis was about the financial impact. At the time I was working for a large professional services firm with a good salary and career prospects. Having studied accountancy part-time for nine years while raising two children on my own, I was determined not to give up everything I'd worked so hard for. I was close to realising my goal (since achieved) to sell the old matrimonial home and buy a low-maintenance townhouse nearer the city.

The type of work I was doing was demanding at the best of times. But at the time of diagnosis the firm was in the process of a large merger and there was a lot of tension and uncertainty about status and future prospects in the merged firm. I was lucky that under my employment contract I was entitled to income protection policies.

I immediately informed the firm of my diagnosis to ensure that my entitlements were protected. This proved to be a two-edged sword. From the moment I advised the firm of my diagnosis, I was never going to be given the same opportunities for promotion, career enhancement, salary increases and bonuses. The discrimination was subtle and difficult to prove, and although I don't think there was any deliberate intention to disadvantage me, it resulted in my being quietly slipped sideways without any real consultation.

About four years after my diagnosis, a claim was finally made by the firm for a partial benefit under one of the income protection policies, and I was able to work reduced hours. The difficulty was that my job was not resized and the promised assistance of another staff member to delegate the surplus workload did not eventuate. I had to train a more junior staff member and compete with others for his services. I was also well down the pecking order for diminishing secretarial services.

It wasn't until after I had resigned my position three years later and was finalising my claims under the income protection policies that I found out about the need for the involvement of an occupational physician (independent medical practitioner). The insurer required a report from one confirming that I was unable to work in terms of the definition in the policies. While I'm very grateful that the policies were available to me and my claims were ultimately successful, the sleepless nights, extra hours of work, the worry and anxiety, and the legal costs to support my claim could all have been avoided if I had been able to access a copy of the insurance policy in the beginning. Instead, I was told by my employers that as I wasn't a party to the policies (it was a group insurance scheme) I wasn't entitled to a copy. The only information I had was the general blurb on the group insurance scheme given to staff on joining the firm. This made no mention that an occupational physician had to be involved. Because of the progressive nature of Parkinson's, it was always going to be a matter of opinion as to when the point had been reached that I was no longer able to work.

An occupational physician could also have ensured my job was properly resized when I started working part-time and that I had all the support reasonably necessary to continue to work as productively as possible. There seemed to be little understanding of what I needed to succeed and to achieve my full potential. I was reluctant to keep asking for assistance, as I didn't want to stand out as a target for redundancy. At the time I did not know enough about the income protection policies to be confident that they would work for me when the time came. The firm seemed ill-informed about the claims process and did not seem to be able to answer my questions fully.

In hindsight, I probably should have sought legal advice about the income protection policies and tackled the employment issues head on at the beginning. I should also have insisted that the change to part-time work and the basis upon which I agreed to it had been recorded in writing and was regularly reviewed to see that it was working as intended. I felt very disappointed that the firm – given its size and status and my seniority and length of employment with them – did not engage an occupational physician at least from the time that I started to work part-time. In any event, I should have sought external help much earlier to communicate my needs and concerns about my future career more effectively.

Using the services of a lawyer

If your employer becomes difficult when you tell them you have Parkinson's, you may need to engage a lawyer who is familiar with employment law. It is even advisable to seek legal advice prior to informing your employer about your condition so that you are fully aware of income protection policies and employment issues.

A lawyer will help you with a range of other documents which you should consider preparing. These are useful documents for anyone thinking ahead to how the future might be for them, regardless of whether they have Parkinson's or not. They include:

✦ an enduring power of attorney
✦ a will

+ a living will or a durable power of attorney for health care
+ a family trust.

Setting up an enduring power of attorney is something we all should do, regardless of whether we have Parkinson's or not. An enduring power of attorney can relate either to property or to personal care and welfare. They are two different documents and it's wise to have both in place. You can have two for property, but only one for care and welfare. An ordinary power of attorney gives someone the limited right to act on your behalf, but ceases should you become mentally incapacitated. An enduring power of attorney gives someone the power to act on your behalf beyond any mental incapacity. It's particularly useful for someone with a chronic illness who is concerned about what might happen if their health deteriorates and they are no longer able to attend to their own affairs. Usually, you would appoint a friend or family member, someone who understands you well. You can appoint more than one person if you wish. You might choose one person to look after your property and another to manage your care and welfare. If you became incapacitated and didn't have any enduring powers of attorney in place, it would be necessary to apply to the Family Court. The court would then appoint someone to act as welfare guardian or property manager.

A will takes care of what happens to your estate after you die. At its most basic it says who gets what. If you have any dependants, such as children under 18, your will should name your preferred guardian and any long-term plans for your dependants' welfare. The will should state who you choose to execute it for you, and include any specific requests for your funeral. It needs to be clear enough to prevent family disputes, though this isn't always possible.

A living will lays out your wishes over what measures you want or don't want taken to prolong your existence, should you be unable to decide for yourself. An enduring power of attorney for health care appoints someone you trust to make decisions for you when you are in the process of dying. I preferred the living will which ensures that my wishes are enforced. This felt important to me after I was diagnosed with Parkinson's. Many people don't want to live if reduced to a vegetative state. A living will allows you to maintain that responsibility for yourself, no matter what. Make sure you discuss this with your family; it is important that they understand and respect your wishes.

Your lawyer will also assist you if you wish to set up a family trust. The purpose of a trust is to protect your assets for your beneficiaries.

To ensure the legality of these documents they must be signed by a witness and a lawyer.

Government support

Once you begin to have difficulty continuing to work, speak to your doctor about what income support is available and whether you qualify. You could be entitled to supplementary income support or a disability allowance, but entitlements will vary depending on your country of residence. Your local Parkinson's Society will be able to provide specific information about government financial support and advice that is relevant to where you live. Contact the relevant government department and explain your circumstances. They will send you a form to fill out and return.

The form generally requires personal information, such as your address, age, personal tax number, marital status, employment history, income, assets (both cash and non-cash), your expenses, relevant invoices and receipts, a copy of your income tax return, and your medical practitioner's report. It will seem very intrusive, as they will want to know full details about your income and assets, as well as those of your spouse. The relevant government agency or office will usually help you complete the form if necessary. The office will review your application and get back to you.

You will then be given the name of an occupational physician (an independent general practitioner) for a medical check. Remember to insist on one who understands Parkinson's. Once the diagnosis and inability to continue in employment is confirmed, you will receive a further letter from the government agency providing you with a number, and informing you that you are now a sickness or disability beneficiary. It's worth keeping in touch with your case manager, as there may be further entitlements, such as a disability allowance, or help with medication costs, housekeeping and other expenses. If your claim is turned down, find out why. It may be a simple mistake and worth lodging an appeal.

When I felt no longer able to work, I discussed with my doctor whether I should go onto a benefit. She was kind enough to explain the process to me, but I felt humiliated applying for and accepting a supplementary benefit. The following year I received a letter reviewing my benefit and asking me to have a further medical check with the same independent physician. I did this, but was pleased a month later to turn 65 and begin receiving the government pension. Somehow this felt better.

A financial planner

Independent financial advice can help you analyse your financial status and focus on your financial priorities – both of which will probably change as your Parkinson's progresses. You can seek advice from a free government budgeting service; or from a financial planner in a private business, if you can afford to.

Choose your advisor carefully, preferably someone who comes with some recommendation. Most importantly, check their qualifications and whether they are members of a recognised professional association of financial planners. Explain your circumstances and inform them as much as possible about Parkinson's. They can advise on investments, family trusts and planning strategies. Mostly, they can help with advice that removes some of the stress you might feel from trying to manage on your own, yet at the same time enable you to continue to feel independent. I also suggest an excellent website that offers advice on most things to do with managing your finances: www.sorted.org.nz.

Changing future plans

▶ *Dave and his wife Ann thought they had their retirement well planned, but then Dave's health problems changed everything. At the time Dave was diagnosed with Parkinson's he had an MRI scan, which proved to be a lifesaver because a meningioma (brain tumour) was discovered behind his right eye. The tumour was surgically removed and Dave took sick leave.*

There was little anxiety or doubt on my part that my job was secure. At the time of diagnosis I was the retail development manager for a large international food company. Nine months later I felt I had to tell them that I had Parkinson's. They could not have been more supportive. I had been anxious about their reaction but my concerns were groundless. They largely left it to me to manage my workload. At no time was my salary in question, which I took as a compliment to my ability and my dedication to the company.

My manager actively encouraged and supported me to plan for an early retirement and move to consulting, which made for gradual transition from full- to part-time work, and eventually to retirement. Everyone I associated with in my work environment could not have been more supportive. I now continue to work part-time as a consultant to the architectural companies who do my old company's design work.

In terms of financial planning for the future, we were fortunate to have several things in our favour. My wife has a background in education. She spent 15 years as a Specific Learning Difficulties (SPELD) tutor, five of them as director of tutor training. Her private pupils provided a supplement to our income when our children were at school and university. As a result of being a senior executive, I received a salary in the top 2 per cent bracket. I invested modestly in equities and took up all staff share options offered. We cashed up our equities when we felt concerned that the market was overheating and invested in a property. The longer term planning at that stage was to build a new rural home for our retirement and to rent out our current city home.

The Parkinson's diagnosis came when the building programme was one third completed. After a nine-month pause while we sorted out the tumour operation and Parkinson's diagnosis, our retirement home was completed. Because of our changed circumstances, we decided to lease the new house while we worked out a viable retirement plan focused on the reality that family and support services are in the city. We then sold the leased rural property, which provided us with an investment income to supplement superannuation.

We thought it prudent to involve financial planners at this point. The sums involved, and my declining ability to manage, meant that we would need professional advice.

My advice would be to plan ahead and have sound goals in place. Most of our planning was done before the Parkinson's diagnosis, at which point it was a case of rewriting/adjusting the plan to suit. We were asset rich and cash poor at retirement (and mortgage free). The revised plan altered the balance. In terms of insurance, we had very minor sums.

Our prudent conservative approach has left us financially comfortable with a debt-free home. We live modestly, which enables us to travel overseas every two or three years.

Insurance

Insurance is the only purchase that is made because we might need it at some stage in the future, which is why many people don't bother. It's a gamble – one that is expensive to maintain, but even more costly to be without if needed. If you have health, life or any income protection insurances prior to a diagnosis of Parkinson's, maintain them. You will not be entitled to the same cover should you wish to extend your policy or move to a new insurer.

The pre-existing conditions clause nearly always limits or eliminates benefits under the insurance policy for medical conditions existing prior to the commencement of the policy. A pre-existing condition is usually defined as any medical condition that has required treatment six months prior to the policy being taken up. Even a consultation with your medical practitioner is defined as treatment.

If you are a member of a group or company income protection insurance or health scheme, notify the person who manages the scheme that you have Parkinson's and keep them advised of your situation. They will probably require a certificate from your medical practitioner or neurologist. They may also require an opinion from an occupational physician to determine your capacity to work. Don't be shy about checking the background and knowledge of the nominated occupational physician; they may not have much experience in neurological conditions and you might want to request a change.

If you're self-employed, you may be one of the few individuals who have joined an income protection scheme. This is sometimes called disability insurance, as it covers you for a period when you may be unable to work because of sickness or accident. My husband used to have it when he was younger, but we don't have it now. Like most insurance schemes it costs more as you age, and it is the expense that puts most people off.

You can still take out health insurance or health travel insurance. Just remember you will be covered for everything except your pre-existing condition. It's also important to discuss with your motor vehicle insurance company any change in your health that might affect your driving.

Driving

If your employment requires you to drive, your Parkinson's shouldn't make a difference for quite some time. However, when you renew your driving licence you will have to declare any medical condition. If you have a commercial licence, you will probably be required to obtain a medical certificate to prove you are still fit to drive.

The range of impairment to the Parkinson's brain can extend to the executive function, which is our ability to plan, predict and multi-task – all necessary abilities to utilise when driving. I don't think I have experienced any loss of executive function so far, but there have been occasions when I've stopped driving through necessity (mostly because of dyskinesia, tremor, or blurred or double vision). Many people with Parkinson's continue driving for years after diagnosis. Because dyskinesia causes involuntary twisting movements, it can create havoc when you are behind the wheel. Your foot surges on the accelerator and your hands are unsteady. You are out of control. If you have dyskinesia, don't drive. It's far too dangerous.

Double vision can occur with Parkinson's because of loss of dopamine. Dopamine loss also slows the muscle response needed for normal scoping from side to side and for focusing from short to long distance, so these actions are no longer involuntary. I have experienced moments when I've felt as though I had to pull focus manually, and this obviously slows the rapid visual response required to drive safely.

Another common vision problem that may affect your driving is the loss of spatial awareness. It's harder to judge whether there is room to park, and moving through narrow spaces is a challenge.

Driving requires you to multi-task – for example, when you approach an intersection you have to look all ways, beware of pedestrians, keep your foot steady, turn the wheel and accelerate.

Those of us with Parkinson's may no longer find it easy and hesitation and panic can take over.

Be responsible. If these problems are becoming more frequent, think seriously about whether you're still a safe driver. Deciding not to drive will be a difficult decision to make. It may be a blow to your independence and it may also be the end of your employment. But the best thing you can do is to know when to stop driving.

—⚬⚬⚬—

CHAPTER 9

Coming to Terms with Parkinson's

When I was first diagnosed with Parkinson's disease, my son gave me a copy of *Lucky Man: A Memoir* by Michael J. Fox. It was reassuring to read how, like most of us with Parkinson's, this famous actor had progressed through the various stages of emotional response from grief to acceptance, and to know that he too had experienced what I call the 'I-want-to-know-now syndrome'. While a need for clear answers is understandable, Parkinson's disease unfortunately isn't that simple. There is no clear path or progression, no way of knowing what to expect. This is what makes it so hard to grasp at the time of diagnosis. How can you come to terms with something so vague? Accepting this unpredictable predicament is the first hurdle.

A sense of acceptance

▶ *It took me some time to accept Parkinson's as part of me. Apparently, I had this progressive disease that would eventually immobilise me, but no one could tell me when. There was no time line of events. I was stuck dreading the worst, without knowing how bad it might be, or when it might be that bad.*

One day I read an article about a hypertension medication that could cause Parkinson's-like symptoms. I had been taking this medication for quite some time. Perhaps I didn't have Parkinson's after all.

During the past months our company had been working on a documentary about the return to New Zealand of the remains of the French Catholic Bishop Jean Baptiste François Pompallier, who arrived in New Zealand in 1839. Because he had been so loved here, particularly by the indigenous Maori, his remains had recently been disinterred from France and flown to New Zealand to be laid to rest in the tiny church at Motuti on the edge of the Hokianga Harbour in Northland.

Early on a June morning, we drove from Opua in the Bay of Islands through low-lying fog towards the Hokianga Harbour town of Kohukohu, which in Maori means 'fog, fog' (where the fog comes twice). That's what happened when we were there; the fog cleared in the early morning, then slunk back to lie over the town again until the sun chased it off.

Just before Kohukohu is Totara Point, the place where Pompallier celebrated his first mass in New Zealand. High above the dispersing fog, a grassy promontory stretched out over the tidal estuary now filling with the steel-cold grey of the incoming tide. A temporary flax whare (Maori house) had been built near the outer edge of the grass. Locals and visitors from around the Pacific were gathering for a blessing of this historic place.

The priests sheltering from the foggy damp under the flax roof of the whare took turns to speak in Maori, French, English and Latin; the hymns were those Pompallier had translated into Maori so many years before.

Many of the congregation were moved to tears, which mingled with the droplets of fog on face, hair and shoulders. A local priest talked of the spirituality of the Hokianga, and how strange and wonderful things happened here.

The sun came out as the service ended and we walked down the hill in silence. From this point Pompallier's remains were to be transferred onto a ceremonial barge and carried to a settlement at the head of the harbour. I was to drive around and meet the barge as it was escorted by waka (Maori canoes) to the landing.

As I drove alone on the winding road above and sometimes away from the harbour, the spell of the morning remained with me. Strange things happen here, the priest had said, and I believed him. I knew then that here was where I would know for sure whether or not I had Parkinson's.

I decided to stop taking my hypertension medication to see if the Parkinson's symptoms would go away. For the next four days that we remained in the Hokianga I took no pills, and the tremor stayed with me. When the time came to return home, I knew without a doubt that I had Parkinson's. I also knew that, like my fine hair and small feet, I would get along with it.

Family matters

We can become so immersed in our own response to the diagnosis that we forget that our family might be hurting too. Recently, my son mentioned that the father-in-law of a friend of his had Parkinson's, and at the time of diagnosis a Parkinson's field officer had visited the house and spoken to the family about the condition. My son wanted to know why I had never offered my family such an opportunity. This question stunned me. I realised I'd spent years shutting my family out of the experience I was going through. I'd assumed because it was me who had Parkinson's, the problem was mine. It hadn't occurred to me that my family might also need support or that they too could benefit from such a meeting. I never asked the question.

I see now I was not the only one in need of support; my children and my husband needed it too. I was quietly grieving for my own loss, oblivious to the fact that they too had to get used to the loss of the strong, able wife and mother I had always striven to be.

Understanding Parkinson's is useful for your family as well as you. It helps you all feel more in control. Your family can take an active role in helping you manage your symptoms, so do consider including them in consultations with your specialists if they wish to support you in this way.

Every family will respond in a different way to dealing with their loved one having Parkinson's. When Judith, a member of my support group, mentioned that she had apologised to her family for having Parkinson's, I was surprised. It had never occurred to me that I should say, 'I'm sorry I have Parkinson's.' 'Sorry' is such a loaded word, but in this context it means that I am regretful – not apologetic – regretful that I am not the person I used to be physically; that I can't do what I used to be able to do; that I need help and find it hard to ask; that I haven't helped those closest to me know when I need support and how they can best help me. Too often we remain silent and make assumptions, and for that I am also sorry.

Be gentle on yourself

Even when you've come to understand and accept Parkinson's, some days will be better than others. Feeling sad, discouraged, frustrated and apathetic is perfectly normal. Some days you feel so exhausted you think you'll never be able to do anything ever again. Be kind to yourself on days when you feel like this. Don't keep pushing yourself beyond your limits; go for a walk or some other gentle exercise, read a book or take quiet pleasure from talking to a friend.

Remember it is okay to talk about Parkinson's; explaining is not the same as complaining. And it's okay to ask for help, too. Being such an independent person, I always hated the thought of relying on others. Now it's time for me to learn to ask for help when I need it. It's not a matter of giving up and letting go, but of knowing when to share. I realise that in choosing not to ask for help I'm not allowing others to feel good by being useful. It's still okay to say no when you don't need help, but phrase it carefully; for example, 'No thanks. I value your help, but this time I can do it by myself.'

Dealing with a sense of loss is a big part of having Parkinson's – loss of health, career, ability, confidence, and sometimes even your relationship with your partner. Every one of these is a major loss, and we can't help but grieve for them. Elisabeth Kübler-Ross, who wrote the ground-breaking book *On Death and Dying*, identifies five stages of grief: denial, anger, bargaining, depression and acceptance. The loss of good health is like a small dying and is something to be grieved for. Unless we move through this process towards acceptance, we can remain angry and sorry for ourselves. If you are finding it hard to deal with mixed emotions as you come to terms with having Parkinson's, it might be worth seeking out the help of a therapist who specialises in grief counselling.

Dealing with a sense of loss

▶ *John was only 43 and was married with four children when he was diagnosed with Parkinson's. He was also one of the world's top athletes. In 1975 he broke the world record of 3 minutes 50 seconds for running a mile. He won gold in the 1500 metres at the 1976 Olympic Games in Montreal, and went on to become the first man to run one hundred sub-4 minute miles. In total, he won over 750 races, and competed for over 20 years internationally. At 43, John Walker was still winning races and in demand for sporting events around the world.*

And then John's Parkinson's was diagnosed. He had noticed symptoms about three years previously. His coordination hadn't seemed quite up to scratch; he'd had mood changes and felt a stiffness in his body that he'd not experienced before. He didn't know what was wrong, but knew there definitely was something wrong. His doctor suspected a brain tumour, and sent him to see a neurologist for a second opinion. Because of the seriousness of the consultation, his wife Helen went with him.

When they were finally told of the diagnosis, they couldn't believe it. Both felt shock and disbelief. How could this be? There was no history of Parkinson's in the family, and John was so fit. He knew nothing about Parkinson's. The impact was devastating. As John explains:

I honestly don't know how I moved on from being depressed in the first few years. I think because my life was busy and a lot was still expected of me, I did not have time to dwell on myself. I had a young, busy family that I relied on a lot, and a business to help run. I told only a handful of people – obviously my family and a few close friends and work associates, and did not go public for several years. But then I had a phone call from a television presenter threatening to make it public. I had really wanted to do this in my own time, but was forced to make a statement to the press. The news of my illness quickly spread worldwide, and I tried to avoid the publicity as much as possible. I didn't want to be defined by having Parkinson's or be a martyr for the cause.

My wife and I had purchased a retail business selling equestrian equipment just before I was diagnosed. The business proved to be a constant in both our lives through the turmoil of those first years, and it has neither helped nor hindered my dealing with Parkinson's. It is just something we do as a day job.

As John came to grips with the change in his physical abilities and the brutal way that Parkinson's had ended his athletic career, he slowly began to feel he had the depression under control and began to take a new interest in the world. He was asked to stand for a local city council by a resigning member, a role he has now held for nearly ten years, and is more involved than ever.

He chairs the community development committee and has recently been able to employ his sporting hero image to establish funds and launch an initiative to get youth off the streets and onto the sports field. It is called the Find Your Field of Dreams Foundation and offers free after-school organised sports programmes and night-time sports at local parks. John hopes the foundation will become a nurturing system for young athletes. In a recent television interview, John said he'd give back all of his medals for good health.

Life goes on

Part of the acceptance of Parkinson's is the realisation that, even though the diagnosis has changed your life forever, you can still keep on doing the things you've always enjoyed with your partner, your family and your friends. Even if you feel unable to work full-time, you can work part-time, get involved in voluntary work, or just do things for sheer pleasure, like caring for children or grandchildren.

Think of all the things you'd still like to have a go at – writing, sculpting, photography. Don't be afraid to stretch yourself – if you want to hike one of the great tracks, do it; if you want to climb a mountain, do it; if you want to travel, do it. Don't let Parkinson's restrict your life.

You'll be surprised how your body can perform when stimulated by a trip, either at home or abroad. But don't be surprised by how long it may take to recover afterwards.

Managing travel

▶ *Judith is a life and business coach and frequently travels overseas. In every aspect of her life she utilises her strength and wisdom. Since diagnosis, she has taken up painting and is now a successful exhibiting artist. But her Parkinson's has not impaired her love of travel, and here she shares some of her travel experiences and tips.*

I have just returned from three weeks overseas on a non-stop ride. We took a 12-hour flight from New Zealand to Los Angeles, had a two-hour stopover in Los Angeles and then flew on to Vancouver, which took another three hours. We stayed there for ten days, played golf twice, and then went up to Whistler for four days. I painted during the day, cooked dinner for six one night, and went out other nights.

Back in Vancouver we stayed with relatives and friends, and then were off to Baltimore via Chicago. We were delayed in Vancouver and were late arriving in Chicago. We had only 15 minutes to catch the plane to Baltimore – we made the flight, but our bags didn't. We had three days in Annapolis, then went on to New York for another three days. All this was topped off with a six-hour flight back to Los Angeles, and a 12-hour flight back to New Zealand.

How did I do it? I believe it was through determination and organisation and by staying calm enough to save energy. I planned very carefully in advance, checking out hotel accommodation, maps, weather and restaurants online. I joined every VIP scheme I could for rental cars and hotels. It cost nothing extra, yet we got priority service. I made sure I had enough money at all times for tips, and used porters where possible. We got upgrades wherever we could, and used airport cars instead of cabs for a flat-rate ride in rush hour.

During the trip I wore comfortable shoes with enough room for swollen feet, and I carried plasters in case of blisters. I used a saline nasal spray on flights to keep my nasal passages from drying out.

When you're travelling, don't be afraid to tell people you have Parkinson's. They love to help you when you have something like this, and will often offer you the best rooms and service, even if they are not quite sure what it is you have.

If you are travelling internationally remember to take your medication every four hours during the journey. Once you arrive at your final destination (a new time zone), adjust your medication to your normal schedule.

Setting new challenges

▶ *Judith had her travel schedule well sorted, but for Cathy it was a case of literally jumping in at the deep end when she heard about an Outward Bound adventure course for people with Parkinson's. Cathy decided to put herself to the test.*

It was the end of summer when I decided to test my survival rate on a week-long Outward Bound course. The first day I learned what was going to be the toughest part of the course – waking up in good humour at 5.30 every morning. What made it doubly hard was the lack of sleep because of the 'chainsaw orchestra' provided by my 14 snoring bunkroom mates. I think I showed enormous restraint in not throwing a few guided missiles during the night.

We were all Parkinson's battlers (I won't use the term 'Parkinson's sufferers' as it has too many negative connotations). We had Parkinson's with varying degrees of severity, and we'd gathered together for our own personal journey.

Cell phones, books and iPods were taken from us on arrival, thwarting any plans I may have had of a nice quiet interlude hiding in a corner to lick my wounds and feel solitary. They were ready for us and presented a punishing regime of daily physical and mental challenges to instil positive reinforcement and self-discipline, and take us out of our comfort zone.

I wondered how I would cope with these activities. I was not at all sporty. I had never been a 'runner', and avoided swimming in cold sea water, let alone at 6.30 a.m. The shakes I had abseiling down the cliffs were certainly not Parkinson's-induced! But as the week progressed I slowly realised that to survive here you didn't need to be sporty.

Team-building, especially morale-building, was the real focus; I came to see how it effectively blocked any thoughts of self-pity. We learned to trust one another and allow others to help us when we needed help. Through humour, a genuine concern for each other evolved.

We were given the tools to improve our self-confidence and keep pushing those boundary lines. At the same time, we were able to recognise our limitations and avoid becoming a danger to others in our group.

The result of attending this course was to be honest with myself and not use Parkinson's as an excuse for avoiding doing something I didn't want to do. I have even taken up running after discovering that I enjoy it and could benefit from it for the rest of the day.

I still smile when I recall our group on our day out sailing, sitting becalmed on our yacht in the rain, playing silly word games, and enduring the indignity of having a bucket of sea water chucked over our heads for an incorrect answer.

The 'chainsaw orchestra' I don't miss, but that week of challenges, that week of seeing us all push ourselves a little further each day, taught me a lot about myself and was an affirmation of what I could do with Parkinson's. I knew that I hadn't lost my zest for life, and that was a pretty special insight to take home.

Parkinson's can draw boundaries around us so that we decide there are things we can no longer do. We convince ourselves there's no point in going on a course like Outward Bound, or pushing ourselves in other ways, because we believe we couldn't do it anyway. We have a go because others bully us into it, and the first day we make tentative progress. Yet by the end, we know we can do much more, and that our life hasn't ended because we've been diagnosed with Parkinson's.

CHAPTER 10

Changing Relationships, Changing Friendships

Your life has changed, and it will keep on changing because Parkinson's is ever-changing. Just when you think you have everything under control, some new symptom arrives. Each new problem brings its own set of difficulties and anxieties, sometimes altering the way you feel about yourself and the way you think others respond to you.

Because many of the symptoms of Parkinson's are so physical, they can seriously impact on your sense of self. The arm-waving of dyskinesia, a vigorous tremor, a bruising fall or car accident can all trigger feelings of uncertainty and inadequacy. These feelings are harder to overcome if you live alone and don't have the support of close family members. This is probably when it becomes even more important to maintain friendships. The difficulty is that often the very time when you most need a friend is when you feel least sociable.

Nurturing friendships

Look for ways of keeping in touch with those you can be honest and relaxed with. Friendships that become one-sided, where one person feels they have to put in all the work, ultimately fail. For any relationship to succeed, both sides need to make an effort.

It's great to be invited out, cooked for and entertained, but what can you do in return? If cooking dinner for friends is too difficult, ask them to share a take-out meal, buy in nibbles from a good delicatessen, or suggest you dine out together. Alternatively, invite people over for tea and cake one morning or afternoon, and buy the cake. Have a card or games evening, go to the movies, suggest a walk round an art exhibition, or a visit to a museum or have a picnic on the grass – activities that don't cause stress or require you to be the perfect host. By making an effort to keep up with your friends they'll want to keep up with you.

Meeting new friends if you are single and hoping for romance may be daunting because you're so aware of having Parkinson's. You can't help thinking, 'Who would want to enter into a close friendship with someone who has a chronic illness?' The only possible response is, 'Who knows?'

Long-term relationships

Sadly, the more anxious we become about not having a close relationship and the harder we try to get one, the less likely we are to succeed. There is nothing more off-putting than someone obsessed with finding a partner, whether or not they have Parkinson's. You will have to socialise, but try to avoid situations where you feel too great a stranger, or where the event is too stressful. Use your friends to beget friends by letting them know you'd like to meet someone new. Most of all, don't tell the person you've just met that you have Parkinson's. Get to know them first if you can. They want to go out with you, not Parkinson's. If they ask what's wrong, be light-hearted. You should be truthful, but you don't have to tell them all the details at once. Don't let Parkinson's become the elephant in the room.

The quest for a partner

▶ *David is 49 and has no children. His marriage ended ten years ago, but he and his ex-wife have kept in touch. She's now happily remarried, and David doesn't regret this, though now realises she was probably the woman he has liked most.*

Over the past ten years David has dated many women, but no relationship has lasted for longer than a year. He has tried the dating agencies, the internet and other media. Now when he tells a new woman that he has Parkinson's, he says she doesn't want to go out with him again.

Although he has a very sporty lifestyle, is good-looking, has a home of his own, has a career, and his Parkinson's is not obvious, he is beginning to feel worried about not having another long-term partner. David works from home and beyond his sports activities he feels he now has to force himself to go out and socialise. Sometimes he feels it would be easier simply to stay at home.

It's hard for David because he spends much of the day on his own; he relies on his love of sport to get out and meet new friends. His chance of developing a close relationship depends on whether he meets someone who wants to be with him, regardless of whether he has Parkinson's.

Falling in love is rarely practical, usually unpredictable and often downright unwise; yet it keeps happening. If the romance lasts beyond that first attraction, it has the chance of becoming a true and loving friendship. Once two people have made a commitment, that commitment shouldn't change because of Parkinson's. However, a chronic illness can place strain on a relationship. The chance of the relationship surviving will depend on the strength of character of the two individuals and their willingness to make it work.

Marrying someone with Parkinson's

▶ *Maurice is 63 and was diagnosed with Parkinson's at the age of 54. He took early retirement from his job as managing director of a company with 8000 employees, which was a tough decision. Now he feels less confident than he used to be. Maurice is married to Karen. He thinks his Parkinson's symptoms probably began about 12 years ago. Karen has her own thoughts on this.*

Looking back, I would say that Maurice probably had Parkinson's when I first met him ten years ago. At the time, I remember watching him walk up my hallway and noticing the way he held his arm by his side. It seemed strange, but I assumed it must just be the way he held his arm, and thought nothing more about it.

Some five years later, Maurice mentioned to me that he thought he might have Parkinson's, as he was finding it difficult to write his signature properly. After going to the specialist he phoned me to confirm that it was indeed the case. I felt very sad for him, but for my part, I instantly decided that I was only going to be positive for him. (Maurice can be inclined to get a little depressed about things occasionally.) Maurice offered to take me to the specialist with him on his next visit, which I found most interesting. I found out a lot more about Parkinson's at that point. We both read Michael J. Fox's book *Lucky Man*, which gave us a good insight into what the disease can do as it progresses. The specialist did say to Maurice that he had a mild case. At the time I took that to mean it would never get very serious, but have since found out that what he probably meant was it would take some time to progress.

Two years ago Maurice asked me to marry him. We had been living together for eight years, and I guess it was the natural progression of the relationship. Maurice did say when he proposed that if I wanted to walk away because of his illness, then he would accept it. But my decision was made without giving Parkinson's a single thought. I thought that if I can be of help, both emotionally and physically (if needed in time), to another human being, especially my husband, then there was no doubt what I was going to do.

We don't know how fast or slow this disease is going to progress. Maybe a terminal illness, which could affect either of us, might intervene along the way. What a waste it would be of valuable time together to throw it all away just because Maurice had Parkinson's.

I am sad and disappointed that Maurice and I are unable to enjoy long tramps and walks. We do a fair amount of travel, but unfortunately cannot do any scenic walks. I can do these activities with girlfriends, but feel sorry that Maurice cannot enjoy them with me. We are able to play golf together, go to the gym, and on a good day Maurice can go for a medium-length walk.

I have a good understanding of the problems that Maurice faces, and make allowances for the quiet tone of his voice and lack of speed in attempting various activities. I offer constant positive support and enjoy the life we have together with its very minor restrictions.

I always think of the glass as half full. Many other people have far worse problems to deal with, and while this is not what I would have wished to happen, it has, and we make the most of all the time we have doing the things we enjoy. None of us knows what is around the corner – my approach is to enjoy today and deal with the progression of the disease when it happens.

Changing roles

Like a lot of couples where one partner has Parkinson's, Karen and Maurice have clearly reorganised their lives to suit. They will probably have to continue to do this as Maurice's situation changes. In some instances, adapting to Parkinson's may necessitate a change of household roles. This is not as easy as it might seem, as it involves gender differences and individual expectations, hopes and dreams.

The knack of adapting

▶ *I'm grateful to Roger and Glenis for sharing their individual experiences of adapting to their changing roles since Roger was diagnosed with Parkinson's at the age of 58. They had always planned to travel and enjoy their time together after their children had grown up. Roger worked in IT and Glenis is an accountant.*

One of Roger's earliest signs of Parkinson's was facial masking and dystonia around the mouth, which made his face seem more severe, and friends began asking if he didn't like their company any more. This was very upsetting, and he had to explain to family and friends that these were symptoms of Parkinson's and that medication would help control them.

Glenis has remained positive, but underneath has been apprehensive.

Glenis: I do fear that life will become too much to cope with as more and more of our daily decisions and activities are likely to fall on me. We don't know how fast Roger's abilities will deteriorate, or what the final outcome of his Parkinson's will be. I am not a nurse and I don't want to see Roger lose his dignity. I also fear that I will lose my own identity as the illness progresses, as it is already taking over how we lead our lives.

Roger: Parkinson's has brought us closer together, yet at the same time has brought more challenges into our relationship.

Glenis: I work almost full days – four days doing contract work for another accountant, and I also work from home for some private clients. I feel that it is a good thing for Roger to do some of the household chores and to take on some of the responsibility of the day-to-day running of the house, but in reality he does very little and not much of his own volition. However, he is taking on much more of the cooking and often decides on the menu before I get home.

Roger: I'm quite comfortable with the sharing of the roles between us as circumstances demand, as I always have been. The cooking is one way of doing my share, although my lack of experience shows up from time to time, and my sense of taste and smell seems almost non-existent, which makes it difficult. Other chores often don't get done. Even when I know they need doing, I just don't seem to get round to them and can waste time around the house with no real sense of purpose.

I've always found I'm much more productive when working with people than on my own. I get mental stimulation and energy from doing things with someone else, or even just being around them. I was never a particularly practical person, but being slower and less dexterous now can also get in the way. Even the keyboard and mouse become major hurdles when your hands and fingers are stiff and slow!

Glenis: For support I belong to a Parkinson's working partners coffee group that meets about every six weeks. We do have someone to contact in the Parkinson's Society, if we need to.

Roger: My biggest fear is for our relationship. Of course, I'm fearful of where Parkinson's will take me physically and worry whether I will still be able to be a positive influence to my grandchildren or become an object of pity in the corner. Our basic plans are the same. For Christmas a year or two ago my wife gave me *1000 Places to See Before You Die*, and we're ticking them off one by one.

As for my career, I have been in IT from way back and was a user of the internet way before 'http' was even invented. When I retired I imagined I would build a website to collect the oral IT history while the people who experienced it are still around. Museums of the hardware exist; but it was the software I was interested in.

Now it all seems too hard and the motivation isn't there. I feel I've lost the initiative and motivation; all the things I wanted to do before now seem too hard.

A lot of us with Parkinson's can easily identify with Glenis when she says she fears for her relationship. This can mean many things. We may fear the change of roles, the loss of status, the loss of dignity, or the loss of love in the relationship. So often illness reduces us, and whether single or partnered, we need the reassurance that Parkinson's hasn't rendered us unattractive to our partner or friends.

Intimacy

Desire and being desirable is a human need and a basic precursor for intimacy and sex. Sexual desire often lessens with age. I once heard comedian Billy Connolly talking about reaching 60 and remarking that he used to think going to bed was for sex, but now he knows it's for sleep.

Our sex lives are usually private affairs, and whether or not we have Parkinson's, we're likely to respond differently to questions about sexuality. For some of us sexual desire is strong; for others less so. What turns one person on might just as likely turn someone else off. What we probably agree on is that our mind guides our sexual response, and it's hard to feel sexy when it's the last thing on your mind. How important is it anyway? It's as important as it is to you.

Parkinson's can contribute to a loss of libido, regardless of age. The main problem seems to be the damaged autonomic nervous system, which in various ways reduces the response to sexual stimulus. Saliva and other body fluids diminish, making intercourse painful for both partners. A doctor can advise on the use of gels or even a hormonal cream which should help to reduce vaginal dryness, increase sensation and prevent pain. Men can experience impotence because of illness, depression or anxiety, but in Parkinson's it is mostly associated with the malfunction of the autonomic nervous system to control the blood flow and subsequent constriction of the veins to the penis (necessary to maintain an erection).

We respond to these situations in different ways. A man needs to know that his masculinity is undiminished. For him successful sexual function is important. As many as half the world's population of men over 40 may experience erectile dysfunction at some time, but this is no consolation if it happens to you.

Don't automatically attribute the problem to Parkinson's. It could be physiological or psychological, so it's wise to see your doctor before leaping to any conclusion. Don't try to cope with it on your own. There are many advertised cures for impotence, but it's best to talk to your doctor before trying any.

For a woman, the loss of libido doesn't necessarily interfere with sexual function, but it certainly decreases the desire. Lack of desire may make a woman feel less desirable, which she may already be feeling because having Parkinson's makes her feel less attractive anyway. The dryness in her vagina contributes to her feelings of inadequacy and makes intercourse painful, both physically and emotionally. Once intercourse becomes painful or unpleasant, it can make us less loving, and sexual activity might become something to be dreaded – he gets weary of approaching and being rebuffed, and she feels guilty for not being more responsive. Soon both feel less desirable and settle into an unhappy pattern where the subject isn't mentioned.

Forgetting to be loving in the simplest ways, such as offering simple expressions of affection like a touch when passing, a gentle kiss, a reaching out to your partner, can happen so slowly that you don't even notice. This may occur because you have become so wrapped up in coping with Parkinson's that you forget about your partner and how they are feeling. Intimacy is not just part of the sexual act; it's about friendship, companionship and the bond you have with your partner. These last three are expressed mostly through touch, kind words and small expressions of how important you are to each other. Sadly, depression, anxiety, apathy and concern for ourselves can make us forget the simple expressions of love, particularly when we don't feel particularly well.

If you feel isolated from your partner through a lack of intimacy, it's important to try to talk about what you feel is missing in your relationship and how you would like it to change. This can seem like the most difficult thing to do. The hardest part is how to make it sound uncritical. Indicating the sort of touch you'd like by offering the same to your partner is a subtle way of making a suggestion without having to voice it.

Too often women are afraid that touch arouses their partner's sexual desire, and too often men find it difficult to separate a loving touch from a sexual touch. A pattern develops in their relationship where both avoid touching and reach out only when one or the other feels the need for sex. This is where an initial pact 'not to go there' can help by providing a 'safe' opportunity to express affection without the anxiety that it will be interpreted as an indication of a sexual need.

Once this caring touch is re-established and a better understanding of each other's needs is achieved, it should be possible to discuss touch for sexual arousal. Couples may have lived together for years without discussing such a simple issue as what turns them on. They may both be surprised by what they learn about each other, and what seemed like a threatened activity may become a new game. And sexual intimacy doesn't have to involve penetration.

If it is impossible for a couple to resolve sexual differences on their own, it may be useful to seek a referral for counselling. Much depends on how important it is to either partner, and how honest they can be about its importance. Unsatisfactory sexual intimacy is often one of the toughest problems to broach in a relationship, whether Parkinson's is present or not; but openness, a willingness to talk, a willingness to listen and a shared sense of humour is a start.

Living and coping with a chronic disease can be a lonely experience, whether you have a partner or not; no one else can truly know how you feel. Even if you feel you've come to terms with the diagnosis, your confidence and self-esteem become eroded with the arrival of each new symptom. This makes it harder to offer and accept intimacy. Whether or not we have a partner to help us through these times, we need to put ourselves forward, care for others, make an effort to maintain friends, and spend time with positive people. Sadly for some, the journey through the long course of Parkinson's will test their closest relationship to the point where it may not survive.

Surviving solo

▶ *Judith is 59 and when diagnosed was married with two sons of her own and one stepson. Her 'boys' have been marvellous, but her husband, a doctor, found it less easy.*

Judith's husband withdrew from her to visit his family overseas. After three weeks he returned, wanting to end their marriage of 27 years. This was a very difficult time for Judith. They went to couples counselling, which seemed successful, and for a while their marriage seemed saved, but it didn't last. There were infidelities that she faced head on with courage, and challenges she met with style and bravado and later recited to friends with great flair. Finally, it was too hard and they separated. Judith moved house and set up a new life for herself.

She has a great bunch of friends who are always there when she needs them. They understand and respect her way of doing things, which is usually full on. Judith has made no secret of her Parkinson's condition. She told work colleagues, clients, friends and family immediately after the diagnosis, and feels strongly that sharing what was happening to her allowed others to ask questions and gain a better understanding of the disease, how it affects her, and how they might support her. Unfortunately, Judith also has Type II diabetes, which she controls with diet, exercise and a small amount of medication.

Initially, she felt she got little medical support, particularly from the neurologist who made the Parkinson's diagnosis. She felt she just had to tough it out and grieve a lot. Her nerves were in such a state she couldn't work so she decided to go away on a five-day retreat. She met some very nurturing women who helped her 'find a path to acceptance'. She went on two more retreats over the next few months and sought out some good healing people.

It is important to her that she is a role model for others afflicted with illness of any kind. She has learned that although her life has changed dramatically as a result of illness, it is possible to find the spirit to move forward and contribute in ways she never thought possible. However, to protect her health and well-being, she has learned to say 'no' when necessary. She used to have neuromuscular massage once a week, but this is now unnecessary as she remains pain-free playing golf twice a week. She attends half-hour exercise sessions with a personal trainer twice a week, one session of Pilates and the other a series of exercises to music dealing with a combination of balance, coordination, stretch and strength training. She also has a treadmill and rowing machine at home and uses them most days for short bursts of ten minutes each.

The combination of keeping her body and mind on the move with golf, gardening, painting and working as a life coach seems to be working for Judith. Her advice to someone newly diagnosed is: 'Check out the path to your spirit and let it sing with whatever takes your fancy. Don't allow others to pity you and get you down. Give yourself time and surround yourself with positive people. Find something to do and give out to the world.'

Support for partners and friends

I have no real idea of how my partner has felt during the last ten years. I haven't noticed any change in him or his attitude towards me. I don't know whether he has felt sad or fearful or hugely responsible. I like to think that because of my fairly practical attitude towards Parkinson's he has felt assured. I ask him. He says he feels sad. He's also proud that I've kept working on various projects.

Many places have caregiver's support groups. If you wish to attend such a group, make contact through the Parkinson's Society, or you can always start a group yourself.

If you are anxious about your partner having Parkinson's and you're not coping with these feelings, talk to your partner first. If there are some things you simply can't say because you fear they will be misunderstood, then I would suggest couples counselling. If you have feelings which you don't want to express in front of your partner, then talk to someone from the Parkinson's Society or a private therapist.

Although your partner has been diagnosed with a chronic illness, they are not an invalid. There's no reason why the balance of your relationship need change at all at this stage. If in the future your partner is not coping as well, that may be the time to talk about an alternative sharing of chores and responsibilities.

Some of you may find it hard not to rush in to help or take over when you see your partner struggling, or when they're taking an age to do a simple thing. You may feel frustration at having to wait for them, or sympathy in wanting to help them, or anger because they're making you late. It's important for your relationship that you don't intrude on your partner's independence. This may mean you have to be especially patient and allow them time to put on their shoes, make a pot of tea or prepare the meal. At the same time, speaking as someone with Parkinson's, it is a good feeling to be asked whether you need help. It's even better when your partner or a family member does the vacuuming, or tidies the kitchen, or makes you a drink without the need to ask. You may find later as the condition progresses that the role you have always played in your relationship begins to change.

CHAPTER 11

Developing Your Exercise Programme

The French writer and philosopher Albert Camus once said, 'Alas, after a certain age every man is responsible for his own face.' This may seem an ironic quote for a book on Parkinson's, which may cause facial masking. However, I've chosen it because I believe that the responsibility you take in caring for your own health and well-being will make a difference to the progress of this condition.

From automatic to manual

From now on, bit by bit, year by year, the things you do – walking, speaking, standing straight, eating, and a host of other everyday actions and tasks – will require more effort. Like the change from driving an automatic car to a manual, things you've taken for granted will require more of your attention.

After some years with Parkinson's, it now takes me longer to get dressed in the morning, and just as long to get undressed at night. There are days when I can barely clean my teeth, do up my bra, put buttons through buttonholes, or pull up my pants. It's not that I'm paralysed – my fingers move, my arms move; they just move slowly and clumsily and without strength.

So what do we do? We get up every day and treat it like any other. We do all the things we need to do and more, and we keep on doing them because you don't give in to Parkinson's.

Long before this slowing down starts, you can do quite a few things to maintain the quality of your life. Most of us are typical human beings and live our lives by habit. Once we learn to walk and talk from birth, we take these abilities for granted; we develop habitual ways of doing things, even breathing. Parkinson's doesn't stop us doing these things, but it does make them more difficult and it will change the way we do them. We need to take control from the very beginning.

From now on exercise will be one of the most important things you can do to help slow the progression of Parkinson's and increase dopamine efficiency. It's not simply a matter of running, walking or going to the gym; it's about attending to every part of the body.

The benefits of exercise

My neurologist told me the first thing he would do if diagnosed with Parkinson's would be to join an exercise programme. Your Parkinson's-damaged brain will benefit from physical exercise by getting the increased oxygen it needs to function better. From personal experience I know that it is important for me to exercise each day and I believe this has helped me to stay well.

Exercise won't cure Parkinson's, but it will make you feel stronger, reduce stress, and improve your cardiovascular fitness; if you include exercises that increase muscle stretch and strength, it will improve your mobility, coordination, posture and balance. Don't forget to include exercises for the voice and breathing techniques as well.

The problem is that our Parkinson's body has a habit of slumbering. It needs exercise every day to remind it how much better it can feel. You may not yet have noticed, but Parkinson's has reduced us; our muscles tighten and shorten, our body cramps, shoulders slump, the head drops forward, arms don't swing, feet shuffle, and even our voice becomes small. Slowly, we take on the posture of Parkinson's; all too soon we can wake in the morning, get up, have a shower, get dressed and function all day in this reduced state without really noticing.

The alternative is to be engaged with your physical self. Free your body through early morning stretches, or take a short, brisk walk to get your circulation going for the day. Stretching exercises keep connective tissue supple and prevent it from tightening and restricting movement. You can even begin them before getting out of bed.

I'd encourage you to devise your own exercise programme; otherwise you probably won't stick with it. Some of you may already belong to a gym; if not, now could be the time to start. I'm not a gym bunny and don't enjoy the communal atmosphere, but I have friends and a husband who wouldn't exercise unless they were enrolled with a gym. Unfortunately, most gyms are expensive. If you can't afford one yet still need an exercise programme, enquire about cheaper community exercise classes, or classes organised by the Parkinson's Society.

Take any opportunity that comes along to try other complementary exercise therapies that might help, such as Pilates, yoga, qigong, tai chi (which is said to improve balance), Alexander Technique or Feldenkrais Method. Check them out online, including 'Parkinson's' in the subject line (for example 'qigong + Parkinson's'). You'll gain a better understanding of each system and the benefits it might offer.

A physiotherapist with an understanding of neurological disorders can help you plan an exercise routine that includes stretching exercises, resistance exercises and a cardiovascular workout. You are likely to have the greatest success with an exercise activity you already know; if, for example, you are a cyclist, a dancer or a rower, these are the activities you should continue to do well.

Whatever form of exercise you choose or programme you devise, it's a matter of finding what suits you and your lifestyle best. My advice is to do whatever pleases you, as long as it gets you moving.

Early morning stretches

Stretching can turn a difficult morning into a sunnier one. You will have more energy, move more easily and think more clearly. Find a stretching programme that suits you and make it part of your daily routine.

I've included my own simple stretch programme here, which I do every day on waking. It is based on Pilates and the programme I followed in a rehabilitation gym. These morning exercises have saved me. If I didn't do them every morning, I would be stiff and sore. You can adapt this programme to suit your own needs. In all of these stretching exercises, be aware of your breathing.

Stretching exercises

1   While still in bed, lie flat on your back and concentrate on your breathing; it will probably have been quite shallow during sleep. Place a hand on your stomach and breathe in slowly. Feel your stomach puff up slightly; breathe out with a sigh. Breathe in through the nose and out through the mouth, long and slow.

2   Still lying on your back, straighten your legs and stretch them, pointing your toes away from you. Now push on your heels and point your toes back towards you. Do this a few times to un-cramp your legs.

3   Stretch your arms down to your sides, hold them stiffly and slide them out so you form a T. Extend your fingers out wide, flexing your hands upwards and downwards from the wrist.

4   Raise your legs until they're pointing up towards the ceiling. Stretch them straight, and once again point your toes up and then down. You'll feel the pull behind your knees. Now you're truly awake, get out of bed. (I usually continue my stretching exercises lying on the floor on the carpet, but if you wish, you can do these further stretches later.)

5   Lie on your back on the floor. Align your shoulders, spine, hips and feet. Lengthen the spine to remove any arching at your waist. Make yourself as flat to the floor as possible, hands by your sides. Stretch your spine, vertebra by vertebra.

6   Move your head in a gentle stretch from side to side, but only as far as is comfortable.

7   This is a good exercise for frozen shoulder, a common complaint for those with Parkinson's. Place your arms by your side, keeping your knuckles on the floor and palms open. Slide both arms out and up in a circle until your hands touch above your head. If you feel any soreness, stop at that point, hold briefly, then slide your arms back down to your side and relax. Breathe in as you move, and out as you relax. Repeat this exercise slowly, five times to begin with, gradually increasing to 20 times. Only go as far as you can, but push a little more each day, and remain aware of your breathing.

8   Now for a version of a pelvic tilt to tighten the muscles in your

abdomen. Lie on your back with your knees bent slightly and feet flat on the floor. Tighten your buttocks and abdomen, and flatten your back down against the floor. Hold for a count of five, relax and repeat about ten times.

9   This simple spine relaxation exercise will help lengthen your spine, and is the best I know for easing backache. Lie with your back flat on the floor. Lengthen the spine to remove any arching at the waist, moving your hips from side to side to stretch and elongate your torso. Draw both knees up to your chest level, clasp them with both arms. Stay still or rock gently from side to side. Feel your spine slowly lengthen and relax. Return your legs to the floor and lie flat. Point your toes forward, then back, and relax.

10 This exercise stretches the front thigh and is also good for your abdominals. Lie with your back flat on the floor. Pull your right knee up level with your chest, keeping your left leg flat along the floor. Place your arms down by your sides. Now lift the left leg just off the ground a little way, keeping it straight. Point your left toes out fully and feel the stretch. Repeat with the left knee to the chest and right leg along the floor. Do 10–20 of these.

11 This exercise stretches the back thigh. Lie with your back on the floor with your arms by your side and your legs straight out on the floor. Raise your right leg, bending it first at the knee. Stretch it out straight towards the ceiling and point your toes. Bring your leg down slowly to the floor. Repeat the exercise with the left leg. Do 10–20 of these.

12 Repeat the spine relaxation exercise (No. 9) above.

13 Lie on your right side. Raise yourself up slightly by resting on your right forearm, using your left hand on the floor to balance and support your upper body. Raise your left leg slightly. Keeping it straight, slowly raise and lower it 10–20 times. The raising must be done by the leg muscles. Roll over on the left side and repeat the exercise for your right leg.

14 This exercise stretches the back of the knee and front of the thigh. Lie on your stomach with both legs flat on the ground. Raise the lower right leg until it is at right angles to the knee. Hold briefly and then lower. Repeat 10–20 times, then do the same with the left leg.

15 This is a general leg- and buttock-strengthening exercise. Lie on your stomach, resting your head comfortably on your arms. Raise your right leg all the way off the ground, keeping your knee straight. Hold briefly and lower. Repeat 10–20 times, then do the same with the left leg.

16 Getting the blood flowing to the brain has got to be good for you. If you can't stand on your head, you can try this simpler inversion exercise. Lie on your stomach, body flat on the floor. Place your hands palm down and level with your shoulders. Raise your upper body as if you were doing a push-up, then rise up off your knees so you are balancing on your hands and feet. You should now be in the yoga position of an inverted V, with your knees slightly bent and your head hanging down below your shoulders. Let your head, neck and shoulders hang so your head feels quite floppy. Stay like this for as long as you feel comfortable.

17 Finally, another yoga exercise to relax. From the inverted V position, drop down into a kneeling position. Bring your hands around and back until they are by your side, fingers directed towards the feet. Lower your forehead to the floor in front of you and relax.

Simple balancing exercises

You can add some simple balancing exercises to your daily programme. Try these where there are walls on both sides (a hallway, for example) to fall against if you lose balance. This exercise is doubly difficult if you have a tremor, and impossible with dyskinesia.

Balancing exercises

1 Stretch your arms out to the side and raise one foot slightly off the floor. Hold for as long as you can without wobbling. Repeat with the other foot. If this exercise is too simple, try the next exercise.

2 Kneel on all fours, hands under shoulders and knees under hips. Lift your right arm and extend it forward, keeping it straight. Your tummy should be tightened and your back flat. Once you've maintained your balance, try lifting your left leg as well and extending it out straight. It's not easy, but this exercise will help strengthen your core muscles. Hold for the count of five while keeping your back flat. If you're wobbling too much and can't keep your balance, stick with one limb at a time – right arm, left leg, left

arm, right leg. Once your balance improves, try raising an arm and opposite leg together.

Exercises for the face

I have periods of remembering to do these every day and days of forgetting. We have a mirror in the elevator in our apartment block and I can fit in a few facial exercises on my way down. A mirror helps a lot.

Try a variety of exaggerated expressions. Pulling practically any face at all helps free up the facial muscles, and the variety of the facial expressions and the funny faces you make will also cheer you up. If you prefer something more structured, try the following exercises.

Facial exercises

+ Count to 20 or recite the alphabet in an exaggerated fashion.
+ Suck in your cheeks or move the cheek muscles separately up and down.
+ Open your eyes wide and roll them around.
+ Make a grimace or a grin.

Exercises for your hands

I have arthritis in my hands, and having Parkinson's as well sometimes makes it difficult to tell which is the most disabling. I'm sure the weakness in my arms, slowness of movement and lack of strength is caused by Parkinson's. The pain could be from either, except for the tired ache in my right wrist and arm caused by the constant tremor in my right hand.

I've developed some exercises to strengthen my hands and relieve some of the pain. I used to do these with a soft foam rubber ball, but lately my occupational therapist has provided me with some therapeutic putty, which is colour-coded from super soft to extra firm. I've found the super soft is perfect for me. It's non-toxic and not oily. It doesn't fragment, stain or stick to the skin, and it offers a wider range of exercises than those I've used with the ball.

You can gauge yourself how frequently to do these exercises – do them as many times as you need, and as often as you remember.

Hand exercises

+ **Clenching:** Hold the ball or putty in your hand and squeeze your fingers into a fist.
+ **Extending fingers and wrists:** Put the ball or putty onto a table top and roll it forward with the fingers, feeling the joints stretch. Then do the same with the ball or putty under your wrist.
+ **Individual finger extensions:** Use one finger at a time to push the ball or putty forward on the table.
+ **Finger pinching:** Roll the putty into a rough ball and grip it between your hands using only the index finger and thumb of each hand. Pinch both fingers and thumbs and pull the putty out to form a thread. Roll the putty back into a ball and replace the index fingers with the middle fingers and thumb of each hand; repeat the exercise. Move onto the ring fingers and thumbs and pinch and pull, then finally using only the little fingers and thumbs.
+ **Finger spreading:** You won't need putty or a ball for this stretching exercise. Place your hand flat on a table. Spread your fingers, extending the space between each finger and the thumb, gradually increasing the span from thumb to little finger. This is a good way of extending the whole hand, and is an exercise often used by pianists or typists (which as computer users we've nearly all become).

Resistance exercises

All the exercises described so far can be done in the privacy of your own home. However, the best way to build up muscle strength is by using the machines available at a gym or workout studio. Studies have shown the importance of strengthening muscles through resistance exercises, particularly in the elderly or those with a chronic illness such as Parkinson's, as they are both prone to muscle loss.

Resistance exercises seem to improve the quality and quantity of mitochondria in our muscle cells. Mitochondria are often called 'the powerhouse of cells' as they are able to use oxygen and glucose to produce energy. Because our muscle cells require lots of energy, they naturally have a greater number of mitochondria. The less we exercise, the fewer mitochondria our muscle cells require; the more we exercise, the more mitochondria can be created. It is therefore worth trying a six-month course of an hour of resistance training twice weekly, using standard gym equipment to improve muscle strength. Your strength could then be maintained by continuing simple lifting exercises or working with exercise bands at home.

Cardiovascular fitness

Any form of exercise that develops your cardiovascular fitness will improve the heart's ability to generate energy by circulating blood and oxygen around the body. Aerobics, jogging, brisk walking, swimming, cycling, and using a treadmill or exercycle will all achieve this. The only one of these that appeals to me is brisk walking, which I prefer to do in the park, though I sometimes use the gym treadmill.

I'm inclined to think that exercise is a lot like food, and should be treated with the same good sense. Any sport you enjoy that gets you puffing, whether it is golf, tennis, cycling or hiking, has got to be good for you because it's the one you'll want to commit to doing. And once you're fit, it's surprising how much more you can achieve in a day. You might collapse in an exhausted heap in the evening, but will do so with a feeling of great satisfaction.

Exercise and neural plasticity

The brain has been mapped and observed since the third century BC, but its capabilities remained largely unknown until last century when the rapid progress of technology and science made possible a greater understanding of the brain and its capacity to heal itself when damaged through injury or diseases such as Parkinson's. We now know that the brain has the ability to recover functionality by reorganising itself and forming new neural connections, and that this plasticity continues throughout our lives. In someone with Parkinson's, for example, the dopamine neurons in the substantia nigra may be damaged to the point where movement is severely impaired, but can be performed almost normally if paced by an external rhythm such as an auditory or visual cue. These sensory cues allow the brain to use alternative pathways that 'go around' the damaged basal ganglia, so that movements can be initiated more easily. This is what makes it possible for someone with Parkinson's whose walk has reduced to a shuffle to be able to walk more normally, play a piano or ride a bicycle. Plasticity can strengthen these alternative pathways, so your brain can respond to a variety of auditory and visual stimuli to make movement easier. Music, singing, dancing and even rhythmical clapping have all been shown to provide such stimuli.

Neural plasticity and singing

While dance seems to provide the ideal combination of music and movement, there have been many examples of the power of music alone. Oliver Sacks' book *Musicophilia: Tales of Music and the Brain* has a chapter on Parkinson's disease and music therapy. He includes some incredible psychological observations of the power of music to restore what he calls 'kinetic melody' – the fluency of normal movement. Yet there is no particular centre in the brain that can be labelled 'music'; instead, music utilises a network involving auditory, emotional, linguistic, memory, learning and movement centres.

Because music has the ability to utilise so many centres of the brain, it has become a useful therapeutic tool, especially when a particular area of the brain has been damaged. Music therapist Alison Cooper is one of the founders of CeleBRation Choir, set up by the University of Auckland's Centre for Brain Research. Anyone with a neurological condition is welcome to join the choir. In Alison's experience, 'Music uses many different parts of the brain. To sing a song you have to listen to the sounds, remember the tune and the words, make the sounds yourself, and finally fine-tune it as you aim to stay in pitch. Even if one part of the brain is damaged, it seems the brain can find new ways to produce a song.' This is a perfect example of neural plasticity – the ability of the brain to seek out and form new neural connections.

The value of dancing

If you don't already belong to a choir or attend dance classes, now could be the time to start. There are organisations you can join, like those that teach music and movement, or ballroom dancing classes. Ballroom dancing is particularly good for us; dancing with a partner provides support through the dance embrace and the opportunity to copy the partner's tempo by following their rhythm. We all respond well to external rhythms. When we walk with another person we match our step to theirs, and in the same way we respond to familiar music and dance to the remembered beat.

The Mark Morris Dance Group

▶ *I felt particularly fortunate to experience classes specifically choreographed for people with Parkinson's with the Mark Morris Dance Group. This New York-based school conducts a variety of outreach programmes in their local community of Brooklyn. A local Parkinson's group invited them to provide a music and movement programme for people with Parkinson's. A small group of four began meeting once a month, and now the centre offers weekly classes for groups of about 35 people. John Heginbotham and David Leventhal lead the classes. These two now train dancers all over the US to work with people with Parkinson's. John explains their philosophy:*

Our intention is to create a gentle environment in which to dance. We offer dance as a joyful activity which both plants us in our bodies and endeavours to free us from fixating on our physical limitations. While we sometimes strive for graceful movements in the class, it is safe to move within any degree of it. It is also safe not to move at all, though attention to breathing and breath is always encouraged. The most important aspect of the class is its acknowledgement that dancing is a disease-free activity. The dancing we do in our class is not concerned with therapy; it is an aesthetic action.

For the duration of the class, the dancers are free to move. When that freedom is not taken lightly, the movements which emerge are particularly meaningful. We move our bodies in the service of beauty, coordination, grace, self-expression, physical challenge, foolishness and fun. We move to music, which is extremely important. Music is a key to taking us out of our bodies and allowing us to be free.

You don't need to have been a dancer to enjoy the Mark Morris Dance Group classes, and you don't have to follow the movements exactly, although they are loosely based on the warm-up exercises of professional dancers. You could even try them at home, accompanied by some of your own music. Choose something in waltz time, and preferably a song you know the words to.

Mark Morris dance class

▶ *The class I attended began with us sitting on chairs in a large circle, with one teacher on each side of the circle.*

We began with a breathing warm-up. Still seated, we did arm and hand exercises to open our bodies up and outwards, keeping to the rhythm of the music.

While still seated, our feet joined in – heel, toe and stamping – again in time with the music.

We stood at the back of our chair and worked our feet alone, then incorporated hands and feet to new rhythms.

Away from our chairs, we began to move freely around the room, always keeping to the music.

Our movements became more fluid and dance-like. The music made it seem much easier. It didn't matter if we made mistakes; it was fun. The classes lasted for an hour and a half, and at the end we felt great.

Being part of a group exercise like this is very affirming and the live music is invigorating. But I can't see why you shouldn't try dancing at home – just put on some music and dance.

The dancer with Parkinson's

▶ *Raewyn is a dancer who was diagnosed with Parkinson's at the age of 58. She is keen to learn to teach the Mark Morris Dance for Parkinson's method and provide us with more opportunity to dance regularly. She talks of her experience of Parkinson's as a dancer, and of being in London where her daughter and grandchildren live.*

I'm walking down Friern Road, East Dulwich in London. It's an early spring day with a fresh breeze, but I can feel the warmth of the sun on my back. My walking has started to change, particularly on my right side, which has a tremor and is less responsive. I notice I am leaning slightly forward, taking shorter strides.

On a subtle level I become emotionally anxious. I ask myself why I am walking like this. So I change my posture, bring my nose back over my feet, calm myself (I call it dropping down into my belly), slow my breathing down and pay attention to my stride, encouraging my ankles to flex.

I feel quite different, as though I'm walking like I used to. I was officially diagnosed with Parkinson's disease two years ago. I say 'officially' because I had diagnosed myself the year before.

As a dancer, this kind of observation and physical adjustment comes naturally to me. Using body sensation as a frame of reference for my well-being is a useful tool; observing all sorts of kinaesthetic sensations has now become a habit. I consciously counter the muscular tightening that occurs with Parkinson's by keeping my spine vertical and my shoulders even.

I take time to lengthen my shoulder joints and calf muscles by stretching. You'll find me lying on the floor, sequentially rolling up and down my spine articulating each vertebra as much as possible, or lying on my side, circling one arm then the other to lengthen the muscles on the front of the chest and down the arm and loosen round the neck and shoulder blades – common places that tighten and get restricted.

The length of time to stretch is indicated by the muscles themselves. You can feel the muscles let go and begin to lengthen rather than being bunched up.

I have been trained to teach an in-depth way of observing and tuning into the body called the Skinner Releasing Technique. I now find it a very useful tool for myself. I find body awareness helps in small everyday tasks. I can't cut vegetables so easily now as my grip on the knife is weaker, but if I use a heavier, well-balanced knife and guide the grip and action more closely, it works better, and putting my index finger on top of the knife strengthens the action.

Consciously exaggerating the flexing of the ankles as I walk works the calf muscles in a better way. I can't sustain it for very long, maybe 50–100 metres. 'Standing tall' and using vision to stabilise myself in all that I'm doing helps me maintain my balance and get fewer bumps when moving through doorways and around furniture.

During the birth of her last child Raewyn received a transfusion of bad blood and contracted Hepatitis C. Unfortunately, this was not diagnosed until recently. She was still struggling with this news when she learned she had Parkinson's.

I hope you now see why my neurologist recommended that exercise should be a top priority after being diagnosed with Parkinson's. Without exercise we risk becoming immobilised too soon. Whatever exercise programme we undertake has to be broad enough to employ all our muscles and stimulate our brain. When you are not exercising, you still need to avoid retreating into that small, reduced Parkinson's you. Whatever you are doing and wherever you are, think about how you are standing, walking or moving. Imagine you can see your reflection in a mirror; straighten your spine, put your hands on your hips, tighten your tummy, lengthen your step, lift your feet and walk tall. Be aware of your posture and movements and don't let your body slide into what is easiest to do.

CHAPTER 12

Taking Control, Taking Care

This is probably a good time to acknowledge, in case you hadn't already noticed, that I'm something of a control freak. I like things done my way. I like straight lines and can't bear untidiness – one centimetre out and it's all wrong. I don't trust anyone except myself, even when I've got it wrong a thousand times. So what happens? This same person who strives for perfection develops one of the sloppiest complaints going and has to begin to rely on other people. How about that! Don't get me wrong, I'm not giving up. I've found there are a great number of well-qualified people eager to help, and I will gratefully take up whatever they have to offer. By seeking out those better qualified to advise me I am still taking control of my Parkinson's.

Voice

One of the most important opportunities I took up was to attend speech therapy classes to improve the quality of my voice. Many people with Parkinson's have voice problems. Sometimes one of the first symptoms is that their speech becomes soft and monotone. It's called 'hypophonia' and is caused by rigidity in the muscles of the larynx, vocal folds (cords) and lungs.

Voice is the sound produced by vibration of the vocal folds within the larynx or voice box. The air coming from the lungs through the vocal folds makes them vibrate and produce sound waves. The force of the air pushing through the vocal folds helps determine whether the sounds are loud or soft. When the vocal folds are shortened they vibrate slowly and produce a low tone. When the folds are lengthened they vibrate faster and produce a higher tone or pitch. If you have Parkinson's, the muscles in your larynx can weaken; they pull less on the vocal folds so your voice sounds weaker.

The amplitude of movement in the vocal folds is reduced, making your speech less distinct and your voice softer. This reduction of movement is typical of Parkinson's. It's the same problem we have with our writing, which becomes smaller, and our steps, which become shorter. We need to be more aware of the way our muscles work; we can no longer take their spontaneous actions for granted. The good news is we can use exercises to pull them into line or, better still, seek out speech therapy before your speech begins to deteriorate.

If you have a voice recorder, try recording yourself in conversation with another person and listen to the playback. You'll probably be surprised at how soft your voice sounds, even though you thought you were speaking loudly.

Vocal exercises will help make your voice clearer and louder. It's better to begin these now before your voice becomes too soft. A voice that can be heard is worth all the exercise; being constantly asked to repeat yourself or not even being heard at all lowers your self-esteem.

Ways to ensure you are heard

Before speaking
1   Avoid talking over background noise.
2   Stand or sit up straight.
3   Swallow or clear the throat.
4   Take a good breath.
5   Make sure you can see the face of the person you're talking to.
6   Think 'loud'; be aware of the distance your voice has to travel.

When speaking
1   Use a strong voice with greater use of emphasis.
2   Think before you say anything and know what you want to say.
3   Pause and breathe between sentences, but remain animated.
4   Keep your hands away from your face when talking.
5   Articulate carefully.

When using the phone

Before you pick up the receiver, pause, clear your throat, breathe in, think 'cheerful', and speak clearly.

There are many simple ways to improve your voice. Practise reading out loud, adding emphasis as you speak; be more aware of the pitch and expression in your voice as well as your facial expression. Try reading aloud to a child, and you'll both enjoy the experience.

If you prefer a more structured approach, see a speech therapist, preferably one trained in working with people with Parkinson's. Ask to do the Lee Silverman Voice Treatment (LSVT) programme. It was designed in the United States by a speech therapist and one of her Parkinson's patients. This series of voice exercises is now taught worldwide. I took the course with an excellent therapist and it made a huge difference to the volume and quality of my speech, and also to my confidence – I recommend it unreservedly. Just remember you'll need to keep doing these exercises for the rest of your life. Pretend you're an opera singer. The neighbours won't mind – they'll probably find you more interesting.

Breathing

Breathing isn't something most of us spend a lot of time thinking about; usually our breathing takes care of itself. Yet almost everything we do depends on us breathing correctly.

When we are stressed our breathing can go into overdrive. It becomes shallow and rapid. We 'overbreathe' or hyperventilate, moving too much air through our lungs for our body to cope with. We begin to feel uncomfortable, not because we lack oxygen, but because we have breathed out too much carbon dioxide. Our blood vessels tighten, which can result in chest pain, faintness and exhaustion; our abdomen and chest become tense and we breathe only with our upper chest.

Even without stress, this pattern of shallow upper chest breathing can become habitual. It's commonly known as 'chronic hyperventilation syndrome'. Because Parkinson's makes all our movements slower and smaller, it's not hard to see how this shallow upper chest breathing can become our normal breathing pattern. To combat this we have to be more conscious of the way we breathe.

If you have any of the following symptoms, they could be caused by shallow upper chest breathing:

+ broken sleep
+ tiredness
+ sighing
+ yawning
+ dizziness*
+ poor concentration
+ shortness of breath*
+ faster breathing
+ erratic heartbeats*
+ physical tension
+ chest pain*
+ tightness in the jaw
+ tight chest
+ visual disturbances
+ headache
+ upset stomach
+ clammy or cold hands and feet.

If you have any of the symptoms marked *, consult your doctor immediately. If your doctor thinks your symptoms could be caused by incorrect breathing, you will probably be referred to a physiotherapist specialising in breathing pattern disorders and stress management. They offer breathing retraining and relaxation techniques to help get your breathing back to normal. (You don't have to have a doctor's referral; you can self-refer.) Most specialised physiotherapists are in city practices; if you live in a rural area, ask your doctor, or refer to www.bradcliff.com 'Find A Physio'.

Here is a simple exercise that will help you understand how you should breathe.

Good breathing exercise

1   Sitting where you are now, focus on your normal breathing function. Be aware that your diaphragm moves down as you breathe slowly in, allowing the lower part of your lungs to fill.

2   Now place one hand lightly on your stomach and breathe in again, this time being sure to fill your lungs, in and low, so that you feel your stomach move out against your hand. Think of the lungs as being pyramid-shaped – big at the base and small at the top. The aim is to breathe the air right down into the base of the pyramid. If you breathe to the base of the lungs, the hand that you have placed on your stomach will be pushed outwards to allow the air to fill your lungs. Try it again.

From this point on, try to make good breathing part of your daily exercise and relaxation programme. The following is a simple breathing exercise, devised by breathing specialist Dinah Bradley.

Simple breathing exercise

1   Lie comfortably on your back. Let your whole body relax – face, jaw, shoulders, arms, hands, legs.

2   Place a hand lightly on your abdomen. Breathe out as much air as possible.

3   Breathe in slowly through your nose. Feel your abdomen puff up.

4   Breathe out gently and effortlessly through your nose.

5   Continue to practise, thinking 'nose – low – slow'. The idea is not to breathe big or heavily, but slowly and low. You will feel your body relax as lungs, mind and body become attuned. As you exhale, think of the tension leaving you. As you inhale, think of the energy returning.

Learning this slow nose diaphragmatic breathing is essential for any relaxation exercise and can be most useful for calming your body ready for sleep. Learning the art of good breathing will benefit you in many ways.

Mouth and dental care

The first advice I would like to offer is that you secure a dentist and hygienist who understand some of the problems associated with Parkinson's and the side effects of the various medications. Dental care is important for all of us, but Parkinson's and some of the medications we take can make the mouth dry and reduce the flow of saliva. This makes us more vulnerable to tooth decay and gum disease. Saliva is a natural bodily fluid that has many functions: it acts as a lubricant, has healing properties, cleans food away from the teeth, neutralises acids and restores minerals.

Tooth decay results in bad breath, difficulty eating, swallowing, speaking and pain. Lack of saliva also causes coughing, mouth ulcers, cracked lips and impaired taste.

Saliva can become thicker and stringier and clog in the throat, causing a choking feeling and a need to cough. Because people with Parkinson's tend to swallow less often, it may sometimes seem they have excess saliva. Remember to swallow – it has to become a conscious act.

Artificial saliva products can replicate some of the benefits of natural saliva and reduce the problems of a dry mouth. They are available as solutions, sprays and swabs in different flavours. Some come with the addition of calcium and phosphate or fluoride for extra tooth protection. Dry-mouth toothpaste is also available. Most artificial saliva products can be purchased over the counter from your pharmacist or dentist, though some require a doctor's prescription.

One suggestion I have adopted is to keep a small plastic spray bottle filled with dry-mouth solution or a tube of dry-mouth gel in my handbag to use whenever needed during the day. The simplest solution for the discomfort of a dry mouth is to drink more water. Carry a drink bottle with you if you can when you're out; it's also useful for taking medication if you're away from home.

Make a mouthwash using sugar replacement crystals recommended by dentists such as xylitol or stevia. These crystals are available from dentists, pharmacies, health food stores and many supermarkets. Xylitol is a natural product found in small quantities in hundreds of plants, including corn, lettuce and raspberries. It is even produced by the body and is found in breast milk. Commercially, it is extracted from rice husk. Stevia is another sweetener with similar antibacterial qualities; it is also a plant-derived sugar replacement. Neither has any metallic aftertaste.

These crystals are used in non-carie producing sweets and chewing gum. Most supermarkets stock an assortment of sugar-free gum, and while chewing this gum may not look great, it is good for your teeth.

A warning for those who have choking difficulties: it is probably better not to use a mouth rinse if there is any risk; an alternative could be to purchase a small plastic spray container, fill it with mouth rinse and spray just two puffs directly onto your teeth. If you swallow the mix it won't harm you. An alternative to mouth rinse is an antibacterial gingival gel which is applied directly onto teeth using a clean fingertip or tooth brush.

Dental mouth rinse

1 teaspoon xylitol
1 teaspoon bicarbonate of soda
1 litre water

Mix all ingredients together. Use this rinse as often as you like.

Baking soda or bicarbonate of soda helps restore the pH balance in your mouth. Since I have a highly acidic pH, I use a baking soda rinse to make it more alkaline. Ask your dentist to check your saliva for its pH balance. I prefer not to add a sweetener, as I don't mind the taste.

Dental checklist

+ Use dental floss or inter-dental brushes.
+ Use an electric toothbrush or soft tooth brush.
+ Use a tongue scraper or brush your tongue.
+ Use a gentle, alcohol-free mouth rinse or antibacterial gel that won't damage mouth tissue.

✦ Use a tooth mousse containing calcium and phosphate to remineralise your teeth.

✦ Invest in an electric power water spray that will help to clean between teeth and remove plaque.

✦ Use a 900 ppm fluoride rinse once a week or a 220 ppm rinse daily (especially useful if you have receding gums).

✦ Decrease sugars and sticky carbohydrates, such as breads, crackers, pastas and cookies or biscuits.

✦ Have periodontal checks twice yearly.

✦ Get advice from your hygienist.

Foot care

Since getting Parkinson's my feet have changed. The skin on both feet is dry, my toenails are tougher and need a lot more care. My dystonia has meant my right foot has been overworked, so it has become larger. The continual movement of my right big toe wears out the lining in my shoe and the toe develops calluses. The clenching of the toes on my left foot makes it uncomfortable, and it is hard to find shoes I can wear, other than running shoes.

I have been to a podiatrist, but prefer to care for my feet myself. I use a rich moisturising cream daily (either a good hand cream or one developed particularly for feet) and rub it well into the skin and around my toes. Apply moisturising cream before bedtime, and if you can bear it, wear cotton socks to bed so the cream soaks in as you sleep. There's a bonus: warm feet help you get to sleep more quickly.

Attend to your feet when they are soft and warm after a shower or bath. It will be much easier to trim your nails with scissors or nail clippers. Use a pumice and emery board to remove dead skin on dry areas.

You could try reflexology, which is based on the theory that each pressure point in the foot corresponds to a body organ. The idea is that you can have your feet cared for and receive a medical check at the same time. Whether you believe this or not, I can vouch for the fact that having your toes and feet bathed, kneaded, rubbed and generally pampered will make you feel great all over.

Sweating

Excessive sweating caused by malfunctioning sweat glands is another symptom of Parkinson's. Excessive sweating can stain clothing and cause embarrassment. Effective antiperspirant/deodorants are available; ask your pharmacist what antiperspirant they recommend. Don't buy a deodorant thinking it's an antiperspirant. Deodorants provide a perfume; antiperspirants usually contain aluminium zirconium.

Some prescription medications help stop excessive sweating, but they need to be compatible with your Parkinson's medication. A neurologist or dermatologist may suggest Botox injections to curb excessive sweating by temporarily interrupting the nerve signals that are causing the problem.

Levodopa can colour your sweat and urine. Spray-on stain removers will remove most sweat stains if applied to the clothing before washing. If you're truly desperate, buy underarm clothes protectors which can be tacked onto your shirts and tops. They are available from dressmakers, clothes alteration shops or haberdashers.

Some men complain of heavy sweating on their head and forehead after developing Parkinson's. This usually happens when they're anxious or stressed and can be very embarrassing. It is probably a result of overactive sebaceous glands triggered by the defective autonomic nervous system and can be helped by reducing their stress levels, watching their weight, and using medication if necessary.

Skin care

Both men and women with Parkinson's can develop oily skin, particularly on the forehead and central part of the face and the scalp; the skin on the rest of the body may become very dry.

If the skin on your face is oily, it's important to keep the skin clean and dry. Cleanse with a mild facial soap. Use water-based cleansers, lotions and moisturisers. Water-based formula make-up and oil-free sunscreen are also available. The regular use of an exfoliate removes dead skin, which, if trapped by oily skin, can cause blemishes. Finding a shampoo and conditioner to suit an oily scalp without making the hair dry is a matter of trial and error. You may find it best to shampoo daily with a mild shampoo. If the skin on your body is dry, use a good dermatological moisturiser daily after showering. Choose one that penetrates the skin, as some can leave an oily residue that rubs off on clothes.

If you feel you need assistance with your skin care, see a dermatologist, preferably one with experience in Parkinson's.

Make-up suggestions

Applying make-up, particularly lipstick, eyeliner and mascara, requires a steady hand. Sometimes tremor or dyskinesia can make this simple task almost impossible. Try these ideas to make it easier:

+ Use a lip pencil rather than lipstick on its own. It's easier to control the pencil and get a better lip line. Apply a gloss or lipstick just in the middle of the lips and smooth it around.

+ Use less foundation and make sure it's water-based. Apply a pearl-sized amount and dab on, first to the nose, then to either cheek. Pat it gently around to the areas where it's needed to smooth out your complexion rather than trying to get it all over the face. Don't put it on your eyelids, or on your forehead if that is oily. Place a tissue over the face and blot gently to remove any excess foundation. An alternative to liquid foundation is mineral make-up in a powder form. Because it's applied with a brush it's much easier to use with shaky hands.

+ To apply mascara, tilt your head back so that your eyelids are down, your eyes are narrowed, and the space between the top of the upper lid and the eyelash is greater. This helps prevent getting mascara on the upper eyelid. Don't use waterproof mascara, as it's too hard to clean off if you make a mistake.

Permanent make-up solutions

If you can no longer draw a straight line and find you're applying, removing and re-applying your lipstick, you may find the frustration is not worth the bother. However, if you want to keep using make-up, you could try getting it applied permanently by tattoo. Specialist permanent make-up colourists can apply natural-looking colour as you want it, where you want it – eyebrows, eyeliner, lips. Women who've had chemotherapy or who have been in accidents often opt for a permanent make-up solution. It is worth considering, particularly if you have a tremor. Ask your dermatologist to recommend someone or check around the beauty clinics. Be very careful to check that your tattooist has appropriate qualifications, examine their photo catalogue and begin with something simple such as eye liner on the upper lid. The procedure is not without pain and a local anaesthetic is applied. There is also a strict after-care regime to prevent infection.

Bladder control

Here is a subject most of us don't want to discuss – incontinence. It can happen for all kinds of reasons, such as giving birth, a bladder disorder or old age, or it might be because of Parkinson's. It happens to both men and women with Parkinson's, and if it is happening to you, you should get it checked. It's difficult for most of us to discuss this with anyone. To admit you might have a bladder problem, especially incontinence, can make you feel like a social pariah. If you do have a problem that seems to be getting worse, it is best to see your doctor and ask to be referred to a urologist.

Meanwhile, here are some self-help suggestions:

✦ Drink less. You need only 4 x standard glasses a day.
✦ Reduce caffeine in your diet.
✦ Empty your bladder completely when you go to the bathroom.
✦ Practise the Kegel exercise to strengthen your pelvic floor.

The Kegel exercise for pelvic floor muscles was developed initially for post-natal women, but is now acknowledged as being just as good for men. The pelvic floor muscles are a layer of muscles stretching from the tail bone at the back to the pubic bone in the front. They support the bladder and the bowel and in men help maintain an erection and improve the blood supply to the penis. A very good reason for strengthening the pelvic floor is an improved capacity for orgasm in both sexes.

The Kegel exercise

1   Sit or lie with your stomach, bottom and thighs relaxed. (I prefer to sit and have the feeling then of pulling my pelvic floor upwards.)

2   Tighten the anus without tightening your buttocks, then tighten the urethra, and imagine lifting it and the pelvic floor up inside your abdomen.

3   Now try squeezing and holding the pelvic floor up for ten seconds, relax for ten seconds, then repeat.

At first you may feel tired after doing this only a few times; if so, try several short contractions. By practising this exercise daily you'll be able to build up to 8–10 ten-second contractions with a ten-second rest between each one, followed by 5–10 shorter squeezes.

To learn to do this exercise properly you can go to a private physiotherapy practice specialising in bladder control, or check the possibility of lessons from hospital physiotherapists or your urologist. Whoever teaches you may teach a slightly different system.

The following exercise is the one that I was taught, and it's meant for women. I practised it standing in the shower, for obvious reasons.

Pelvic floor exercise for women

✦   Stand straight, with your feet slightly apart. Place the middle finger of your right or left hand just inside your vagina. Pull in your buttocks and contract your pelvic floor muscles to tighten around your finger. Hold for a slow count of one, two, three, or whatever you can manage, and relax. Don't feel defeated if you can't feel a tightening the first few times; keep trying and eventually those muscles will remember what they're supposed to do. Do this as many times as you can to begin with, and then to the count of 20 a day once you find it easier.

✦   Once you have felt the contractions and know how to achieve them, you won't need to use your finger to check you're doing the exercise properly.

Constipation

Like incontinence, constipation doesn't just happen to the elderly. For most of us, constipation and bladder incontinence are subjects we avoid and wouldn't dream of discussing, even with our best friend. But if you experience any problem lasting for more than a few days, talk to your doctor. Parkinson's can cause constipation by slowing the muscles of the bowel wall, stomach, pelvis and the anus. A colonoscopy is the best way to identify whether there is any other medical condition within the colon.

Once it has been established that the constipation is caused by Parkinson's, there are some things you can do to help your body maintain healthy bowel function. They include the following:

+ Generally increase your fluid intake. (This will depend on your bladder being okay.)
+ Always take your medication with a glass of water.
+ Have a glass of warm water with lemon juice first thing in the morning; add a teaspoon of honey, if you prefer.
+ Include more fibre in your diet. Try adding bran to your breakfast cereal, and have an apple at lunch.
+ Have a healthy cereal breakfast with fresh or dried fruit and a morning cup of tea or coffee.
+ Eat regular meals.
+ Get plenty of exercise. Aim for 30 minutes of aerobic exercise daily, and maintain abdominal muscle strength through abdominal exercises.
+ Establish a bowel routine at a time when you can have the bathroom to yourself and have time to relax.
+ Don't ignore the urge to go.
+ Try massaging your abdomen. While sitting on the toilet, place your open right hand above your navel towards your left side, pressing downwards on that side. Move your hand in a circular movement. Keep the pressure on that left side and lean forward slightly. Allow yourself time.

It is most important that constipation is not left to become worse. If you have tried most of the suggestions and still have a problem, your doctor will arrange for medication.

We've covered some of the ways you can care for yourself, but I do recommend you get professional advice if you feel unsure of anything. Professionals such as those acknowledged here have specialised in their fields of health care; they can make you confident you are caring for yourself as best you can.

—∞∞—

CHAPTER 13

Relaxation

Most of us think of relaxing as watching television, reading a book, or taking a long, slow soak in a bath. All these activities are relaxing, but the sort of relaxation I'm referring to in this chapter is the regular practice of some form of deep relaxation – for example, breathing exercises, yoga, meditation, progressive muscle relaxation, autogenic training or visualisation. During deep relaxation your brain switches off from analytical thinking. Practising deep relaxation exercises regularly can bring about physiological changes, such as a lower heart rate, a lower respiration rate, lower blood pressure and less muscle tension.

Because Parkinson's can interfere with the functions of the organs, glands and muscles, we need to learn ways of assisting our bodies to return to good physiological balance. Developing a habit of deep relaxation for 20–30 minutes each day can help achieve this. You should begin to sleep better, feel less fatigued, experience less panic and have improved concentration and increased energy.

Progressive muscle relaxation

This yoga exercise is excellent if you're having trouble sleeping. You can do it on your own, or get someone to talk you through it. It contrasts muscle tension and relaxation; you breathe in as you tense, and out as you relax. I worked in a hospital for a time and used this to help patients relax prior to surgery.

The following is a fairly condensed version. You can make it longer if you wish by being more aware of each part of the body as you progress through the exercise.

Relaxation exercise

1   Find a comfortable place, either on the floor or on a bed without a pillow. Be sure you're lying quite straight with your arms relaxed and lying out from your sides with palms facing up. Point your toes away from you, then relax your feet and lie comfortably.

2   Be aware of your breathing. Breathe out as much air as possible; breathe in slowly through your nose; feel your abdomen puff up; then breathe out gently and effortlessly through your nose.

3   Once your breathing is slow and regular, begin the progressive muscle relaxation. At each stage of the exercise, breathe in as you hold the muscle contraction, and breathe out as you relax.

4   First focus on your toes. Wriggle them, then contract them, holding the contraction as you breathe in; then relax as you breathe out.

5   Now work on your feet. Wriggle them, contract them, then relax. Let your feet flop and feel the release of tension.

6   Gradually work your way up your body, from the feet, to the calf muscles, the knees and the thighs, alternating muscle tension with relaxation. Be aware of how your lower body is feeling; let the tension go so that your legs feel heavier now and quite relaxed.

7   Moving further up the body, imagine your buttocks pressed against the surface you're lying on. Tighten them as you breathe in, and relax as you breathe out. Do this also with your stomach and pelvis, pulling that part of your body in tight as you breathe in, and relaxing as you breathe out. Feel your hips and stomach releasing their tension from your body.

8   Next, focus on your breathing and your diaphragm. Concentrate on breathing – in through the nose, then slowly out. Feel your diaphragm relax inwardly, letting the tension drain away; your body will feel heavy, as if it could sink into the surface you're lying on.

9   Focus next on your shoulders and any area of tension in them. Be aware of this as you contract them, and then let all pain and tension drain away as you relax.

10   Now wriggle your fingers and clench and unclench you fists. Feel how the clenching of your fingers tenses your arms; contract as you

breathe in, relax your arms, hands, fingers as you breathe out.

11   Be aware of how heavy your head feels against the surface you're lying on. Move it gently from side to side; if there is any pain in your neck, be aware of it, simply noting its presence and move on to your head. Feel how your scalp covers your head and tighten your skin as you breathe in, relax as you breathe out. Scrunch up your forehead and relax. Do the same with your cheeks and allow your mouth to soften and open slightly. Feel your face relaxing, all the tension ebbing away and leaving it calm.

12   Concentrate once more on your breathing, keeping it low, your diaphragm gently rising as you breathe in, then feel the breath pass out effortlessly through your nose. Feel how heavy and relaxed your whole body is, and allow your mind to go with it and relax. Stay like this for as long as you want to.

Managing Parkinson's through yoga

▶ *Chandra is 52 and married. She has three adult children, a large extended family and many friends. She was diagnosed with Parkinson's aged 45, and from that time she has been on a long search to find a cure. Sadly, this hasn't happened, but through her search she has discovered ways to relax and live with Parkinson's. She learned a meditation and relaxation technique in her native India.*

With two other members of the family Chandra and her husband went to Gujarat, then toured North and South India. During the six months they were away they visited two Indian neurologists who confirmed her diagnosis and suggested some Ayurvedic medicines.

During the next two years, Chandra's symptoms slowly worsened. She and her husband planned a return visit to India. This time they travelled south to an Ayurvedic centre in Kerala, where they stayed for 28 days. Chandra says this experience helped conquer her fears and she learned valuable ways of coping with depression through yoga.

In Mumbai they visited a guru who teaches a breathing technique called Krya or Pranayaan, and this more than anything has helped her. Since then, Chandra has visited him in Fiji and spent a further four months of study there. She has adopted a regime which she follows strictly each day in a room she has set aside at home.

She rises between 4.00 and 5.00 a.m. and meditates for an hour. This is followed by 30 minutes of yoga exercises, a calming down, and then breathing exercises for a further 30–45 minutes. She then showers, has breakfast and is ready for the day. In the evening she practises only the breathing exercises. Chandra intends to follow this path of calming meditation and yoga healing alongside conventional medicine. She feels she has found a technique that helps her live with Parkinson's.

Visualisation

Visualisation is an applied relaxation technique that is fairly simple to learn. It can be useful in calming the body and mind in preparation for sleep, or it can be used simply as a relaxation exercise.

It is preferable to do it lying flat on your back somewhere warm and where you won't be interrupted. Allow 20–30 minutes. It's better if a friend or partner talks you through it, but if you have the confidence you can do it alone by thinking yourself through a story. Here is a condensed version.

Visualisation relaxation exercise

1   Find a warm space where you're comfortable lying down. You could use a yoga mat, a rug or carpeted floor, and a pillow, if you prefer. Dim the lights. If you're trying to encourage yourself to get to sleep, it's probably best to lie in bed.

2   Lie flat on your back, legs straight and arms relaxed at your sides. Close your eyes. You're about to go on a mind journey, imagining your body in another location. It is pleasant, warm and comfortable. For example, you might imagine a tropical journey where you're lying on a white sandy beach in the warm sun or under the shade of a tree. Because this is a mind journey, the possibilities are endless. Choose any journey you like. It can be the same one each time or a different one, but keep to the one story during the session.

3   Explore this location with your mind, touching all the senses one by one. Imagine the feeling of the sand or the petals, the water or the grass you lie on. Hear the sounds around you, the swish of the sea and a breeze in the palm trees or just the stillness. Feel the warmth of the sun on your body or the softness of sand under you. Smell the salt water, the sand or the leafy scent of the forest. Be aware of the colours around you, the brightness of the sun, the shade of the tree or flowers, the sky and clouds drifting above you.

This is a mind journey and can last for as long as you choose. The main thing is to keep it pleasant and relaxing, soothing and comforting, safe and simple. You can cease the journey at any point, but preferably at a moment where you have achieved complete relaxation. At that point, lie where you are for as long as you like and enjoy the moment.

Massage

Touch is a powerful healer. Our natural instinct when injured is to place our hands on a wound or rub it. Children instinctively call out for a parent when hurt, wanting to be 'kissed better' or needing a hug for comfort. So it's not surprising that when we grow to be parents ourselves we understand how touch can make monsters disappear, soothe away bad dreams and reassure us that all is well.

From this basic human instinct cultures have developed techniques of touch for a range of bodily ailments; we know these techniques as massage. When you have Parkinson's, massage can be beneficial in a variety of ways. It can enhance our sense of well-being, help release muscle stiffness and local tension, increase joint mobility, decrease inflammation, improve circulation and relieve pain.

Massage techniques vary greatly and the one you choose will depend very much on what seems to help your Parkinson's symptoms the most. The most widely offered massage is a therapeutic or Swedish massage. It forms the basis of most massage treatments. It consists of kneading, stroking, finger tapping and hand pressure. Sports massage removes tension in soft tissues, and may be of use in aiding recovery if you have a fall. It may be deeper and more intense than therapeutic massage. Thai massage is based on manipulation. The body is placed in a variety of positions, your limbs stretched and pressures applied that can be intense. Shiatsu (meaning 'finger pressure') uses gentle finger pressure to adjust the body's energy flow.

Most massages last about an hour and may require you to be dressed or undressed. As with any complementary therapy, it is important to be sure that the person administering the massage is qualified to do so. It is a good idea to talk to friends with Parkinson's who receive regular massage and who recommend their masseur or the clinic treating them.

Autogenic training

The autogenic training method relaxes the body through auto-suggestion. It may also be called self-hypnosis, depending on the trainer. It is said to restore the balance of the autonomic nervous system, lowering blood pressure and slowing the heart rate. Autogenic training can be particularly useful for those with Parkinson's who find getting to sleep difficult. If you think it could help you, look for a therapist, psychologist or a yoga centre that teaches it, as it does require you to learn the method.

Finding a relaxation technique that suits your personality and needs can be a bit like massage in that you have to try a variety of different types to get the right one. And in the end you may eschew all of these for a simple breathing exercise.

CHAPTER 14

·∞∞·

Diet and Dietary Supplements

As someone who enjoys cooking and appreciates a well-presented meal, I remember being appalled many years ago when my father-in-law described meals as a 'refuelling exercise'. He was right, in a way. When he was a young man, a meal consisted of meat and milk from a local farm, and vegetables from the home garden. You worked hard, life was simple, and food was uncomplicated. Halfway through last century our food became complicated. It was processed for convenience and to 'enhance' taste. Nutrients, flavours and colourings were added, and what we now call the Western diet was developed. Some people who have emigrated from Eastern countries have seen their diet adopted by those in the West. However, too often the children of immigrants are attracted to the fast foods of the new country. Sadly, fast food results in obesity and poor health for many.

You don't meet many people with Parkinson's who are overweight. For most of us the problem is actually how to maintain our weight, as both tremor and dyskinesia burn up calories. If you're losing weight, you'll need to eat more.

Weight loss can lead to muscle loss and fatigue, reducing our ability to stay fit and maintain strength and stamina. Parkinson's lowers our immune system, which in turn makes us more vulnerable to infections. But do we need a special diet? I don't believe so. Some of us may have other health problems, such as diabetes or coeliac disease, which require special dietary considerations. What we need is what most healthy people need – a balanced diet that will boost our immune system, aid healing, maintain strength and generally keep us as healthy as possible.

Eating a variety of foods will provide us with the nutritional elements our bodies need. The healthiest way of achieving a correct balance is through a simple diet of lean meat, fruit and vegetables. To maintain our body's pH level and good kidney function, balance protein-rich foods such as meat and grains, which are acid-releasing, with foods such as green vegetables, which are alkali-releasing.

When I eat meat I prefer it to be free-range and, if possible, farm-killed. Food is best eaten closest to its natural form and processed as little as possible. Real food doesn't need to be altered in complicated ways or nutritionally 'created'. Fruit and vegetables are best fresh, but frozen or canned produce can be used. I generally use frozen peas as they're more accessible. I use canned tomatoes, for similar reasons; although they don't taste as good as fresh tomatoes, they are cheaper and easier to use.

Food for energy

When you feel tired it's all too easy to grab an energy bar and fool yourself that you've eaten well, but there are tastier and more satisfying ways of restoring your energy. Try including some of the following foods in your diet; they will help you maintain your weight as well as boost your energy levels:

+ avocado
+ olive oil and other vegetable oils
+ peanut, almond or hazelnut butter
+ dried seeds, nuts and fruit
+ honey
+ milk, butter, cream, ice cream and sour cream
+ cheeses of all kinds
+ coconut cream
+ eggs.

Some of these foods, such as honey and ice cream, contain sugar, and others, such as coconut cream and butter, are rich in fat and so may not be suitable if, for example, you have diabetes or cardiovascular problems. However, we do need adequate amounts of fat in our diet in order to be able to absorb vitamins such as vitamin A and vitamin E. Both are antioxidants and may improve our Parkinson's lack of immunity.

Diet and medication

We know that levodopa needs to be absorbed from our small intestine. Because some foods can delay the absorption, we usually take it on an empty stomach. However, there are exceptions. Some people find the first dose of the day can cause nausea unless taken with a cracker or toast; others who suffer from dyskinesia because of fluctuating or higher levels of levodopa may require food to slow the absorption of the medication. Foods that seem to achieve this best are those that are high in protein, such as a glass of milk, a dish of ice cream or a milkshake.

The reason why proteins may restrict levodopa is because proteins contain amino acids, and these amino acids exist in levodopa as well. If all the amino acids are competing to get into the bloodstream at the same time, the result could be less levodopa being absorbed. We don't usually want a lowered level of levodopa, except when it provides relief from dyskinesia.

Protein-rich foods

The amino acids contained in proteins are the body's building blocks and are essential for the growth of body cells and tissue repair. Protein-rich foods are meat (including fish and poultry), milk, cheese and eggs. However, a protein-rich diet can cause excess acidity. To prevent our system becoming too acidic, we need to balance our protein intake with energy foods (such as carbohydrates), fats and alkali-releasing green vegetables. If we cut down on our meat intake or eat a vegetarian diet, we need to combine plant proteins by mixing whole grains, nuts and legumes.

'Legumes' is another word for pulses, which are peas, beans and lentils. They have been used as food for thousands of years, are high in protein and carbohydrate, and low in fat. They include chickpeas, lentils, lima beans, kidney beans and broad beans (or fava beans). Broad beans contain a natural levodopa, but not enough to make them a replacement for medication. (Some people have an allergic reaction to broad beans known as favisim, but I'm sure you would know if you had this inherited problem.) Dried beans, particularly soy and kidney beans, need to be soaked for up to 12 hours before cooking. They must then be well rinsed and thoroughly cooked to remove toxins before they are eaten.

Carbohydrates

There is a theory about carbohydrates and Parkinson's. Carbohydrates increase insulin emission, which can lower amino acids in the blood. Theoretically, this lowering of competition in the blood allows more levodopa to travel to the brain. Because carbohydrates increase insulin emission, they are also the main source of energy in our diet and are particularly important for those of us who find it difficult to maintain weight. In the mornings we need energy and levodopa to free up mobility. This would suggest we should have a carbohydrate breakfast. However, should an increased levodopa cause dyskinesia, we may have to balance our breakfast carbohydrates with protein.

Choose fresh and free-range

When I discuss dietary requirements, I'm reminded of my grandmothers, both of whom baked their own wholegrain bread and churned cream from the farm into rich, yellow butter, exquisitely rolled into small balls ready for the table. I'm not about to bake my own bread or produce butter in my city kitchen, but I can choose wholegrain bread from the local bakery, and organic butter. I can bake cakes and biscuits from wholegrain flour, butter, free-range eggs and raw sugar or honey. I can get all the complex carbohydrates, proteins, fats, vitamins and minerals I need from combinations of whole grains, nuts, seeds, eggs, butter, cheese, milk, fruit and vegetables. And I don't have to read the ingredients list on any of them.

Some fruit and vegetables are shipped long distances and may have been sprayed with chemicals to keep them fresh. Have a go at developing your own vegetable garden. As well as making economic and ecological sense, the fresh vegetables you harvest are good for your health, and gardening is therapeutic. Enjoy the range of foods introduced by various ethnicities. Try to buy only in-season fruit and vegetables, and wash them prior to storing or cooking. Buy whole foods without additives, free-range everything, and enjoy variety in moderation each day.

Keeping up the fluids

Don't forget to drink plenty of fluids. These dissolve essential vitamins and minerals, help maintain our blood pressure and flush away toxins. Water aids digestion and chemical change and is necessary for our blood supply and normal bowel function. It's debatable how many glasses we need daily – six or eight is generally advised, but we can include tea, coffee, milk, juice, jelly and soup in our fluid intake. I have a glass of water each time I take my medication. This ensures I have six glasses to start with and helps moisten my otherwise dry mouth, a common problem when you have Parkinson's. You may choose to carry water with you every day in a drink bottle, but be sure the bottle is thoroughly sterilised if you intend to re-use it.

Responding to your body's needs

Be more aware of how your body copes with various foods and drinks. Notice those foods that don't seem to suit you, or cause nausea, flatulence, dyskinesia, constipation, indigestion or headaches. I like almonds and used to snack on them until I realised they were causing flatulence, and sadly I had to give them up or live a lonely existence.

My favourite meal is breakfast. I like porridge; my favourite breakfast is home-made muesli, yoghurt and fresh fruit. When the nineteenth century Scottish writer Sir Walter Scott visited his friend the English poet William Wordsworth and his wife Mary, he reported that they fed their family three meals a day, two of which were porridge. Like the Wordsworths, I could live on porridge or muesli twice a day because I like it so much, and know it's also good for me – oats contain more protein and fat than other cereals and are rich in minerals and vitamins.

I feel so positive about the benefits of my Oat Muesli recipe I'd like to share it with you. It has taken me years to perfect and provides everything I want in taste, nutrition and dietary fibre. It's perfect for people with or without Parkinson's. Give it a try.

The recipe quantities below should last for a week or two, depending on how many of your friends and family you share it with.

Oat Muesli

1 kg rolled oats (or jumbo oats if you prefer)
200 g sunflower seeds
200 g pumpkin seeds
100 g coconut chips (grated pieces)
100 g white sesame seeds (optional)
100 g oat bran
75 g wheat germ
75 g ground linseed
100 g cashew or hazel nuts
100 g slivered almonds
200 g dried cranberries or other dried fruit such as apples,
     apricots or raisins

Preheat the oven to 180°C. Combine the first five ingredients in a large oven dish. Bake for 30 minutes until the mixture starts to turn golden. Turn off the oven and allow the mixture to cool in the oven. Once cool, add the remaining ingredients and mix together well. Store in a large airtight container. Serve with fresh Greek yoghurt, milk, a teaspoon of honey and fresh fruit.

Use this recipe as a guide, if you wish, and modify it to suit your taste and particular ethnic cuisine.

One time of day that your body may need more sustenance is during the afternoons when you feel tired. Nutritional drinks and supplements are available, but I prefer a chocolate milk drink, a fruit smoothie or an ice cream. If you have a balanced lunch of carbohydrate and protein followed by fresh fruit, you should find you don't get so fatigued in the afternoon.

For your overall health and well-being, you might consider eating less meat, which is protein-rich and harder for your Parkinson's system to digest. Vegetarian food doesn't have to be tofu (which can be delicious), nut rissoles (try falafels) or raw cabbage. A well-planned vegetarian diet is healthy, easily digested, sustaining and appetising. It does require more forethought and preparation, but it's certainly not just a plate of vegetables without meat.

More than just food

As you've probably realised by now, food matters to me; I care about what I eat and how it's presented. I enjoy reading about food, looking at recipes and preparing, cooking, serving and eating food that looks good, tastes good and is good for you. I think of meals as social occasions, a time for family or friends to sit down together, share food and conversation, an opportunity to take time out and enjoy the company of others.

But what if some time in the future I can no longer cook? What if Parkinson's affects me so badly that I can no longer cut, chop, stir or whip to prepare, produce or serve the sort of meals I like? How will I cope with someone else's idea of a meal, and what might that food be like? This is something that really concerns me.

I presume my husband would have to cook. When we were married he told me that he saw food as 'refuelling', just like his dad. I know he doesn't think this today, but he still prefers not to cook. It's not that he can't, but that he doesn't wish to. Because I've been so assertive in the kitchen, he has preferred to leave it to me; for years I discouraged him by heaping scorn on his unremarkable efforts. Now it's these efforts that I may have to put up with.

I've told him that men who cook are sexy. I've encouraged him to go to cooking classes and he can make breakfast, lunch and a good salad. I guess it's up to me. If I want to eat interesting meals, then I need to make more of an effort to teach him. He needs more encouragement and my appreciation.

Dietary supplements

Like many people with a chronic illness, I'm interested in holistic health. I have friends who are naturopaths or other alternative healers, and I enjoy talking about alternative approaches and remedies with them. As a result, I have tried various supplements and may try others in the future. The recommendations made here are based on my own experience and may or may not be effective for everyone.

In the twenty-first century the marketing and consumption of supplements has risen hugely. Now there are natural health shops everywhere you go. I don't remember seeing one when I was a child, though our mothers gave us malt by the spoonful and cod liver oil capsules in winter.

Natural health treatments are a multi-million dollar business and international companies are highly competitive; research within these companies is as serious as that undertaken by any medical researchers. Who can say what new discoveries will be realised by graduates and researchers at colleges of naturopathy and the various schools of holistic medicine?

I don't know whether supplements help make you healthier or not. It seems the argument as to their benefit will always be with us. However, just in case, I sometimes take a powdered multivitamin and mineral supplement to boost my Parkinson's-reduced immune system, and a daily omega 3 capsule for my brain and heart.

Since I have arthritis, particularly in my hands, I also take glucosamine and chondroitin. These were recommended by my rheumatologist, who agreed with my taking omega 3 as an anti-inflammatory, though I originally began taking it because I have coronary artery disease and believed it might reduce the risk of a heart attack.

The belief in a product can be so strong as to persuade you of an improvement in your symptoms. This is sometimes referred to as 'the placebo effect' and is commonly noted when a drug is being tested – half the trial participants take the drug being trialled and the rest a placebo; those on the placebo often feel they have benefited from the drug to some degree.

Supplements may work in the same way as a placebo. We can be sure of the benefits of some supplements, although whether we need them is debatable.

The importance of antioxidants

It's impossible to talk about antioxidants without first explaining free radicals; they're the reason we need antioxidants. We're all made up of cells, which consist of molecules, which are in turn made up of atoms. Free radicals are oxygen atoms that are missing one electron from the pair they should have. An atom missing an electron becomes unstable, so it grabs an electron from a neighbouring atom. That atom then becomes a free radical, because now it's the one missing an electron. One free radical starts a chain of free radicals in our body, grabbing electrons from our cells, and doing a lot of damage at the same time.

Some free radicals occur naturally during the process of metabolism, or when our immune system creates them to fight bugs and disease. But toxins such as herbicides, insecticides, UV rays, radiation and pollution can all create free radicals. Some researchers think there could be links between these toxins, free radicals and diseases such as cancer and neurodegenerative diseases like Parkinson's.

Antioxidants are molecules that can interact with free radicals and terminate the chain before important molecules are damaged. Our body has its own defence system of antioxidants, and we can boost our protection by including naturally occurring antioxidants in our diet.

The most important antioxidants are vitamins C and E. I eat plenty of fresh green vegetables and fruit, which contain vitamin C, and nuts, wheat germ and soy beans for vitamin E. I have taken a vitamin C supplement mainly because I thought it would boost my immune system, as Parkinson's is known to reduce its efficiency. However, recent studies suggest that echinacea is more beneficial in helping prevent winter colds, so I stopped taking supplementary vitamin C.

Selenium, a trace mineral, is also an antioxidant, but is only required in small amounts. Brazil nuts are high in selenium; two a day provide your body with all the selenium you need. Because of this, it's best to eat fewer of them than other nuts.

Coenzyme Q10 (CoQ10) is another antioxidant present in small amounts in our bodies, but as we grow older we make less of it. We can get it from nuts, unsaturated oils and meat, especially liver. Because of its role as an antioxidant, it has been suggested as being beneficial in slowing Parkinson's. However, the difficulty of getting a supplementary CoQ10 across the blood–brain barrier means you would have to consume well over 1000 mg a day, and there's no proof that it would help reduce the symptoms of Parkinson's. You can buy CoQ10 from a pharmacy or health store in tablet form, but I would advise you discuss with your neurologist first whether to take it.

Some people with high cholesterol levels, heart disease and diabetes may take statins (lipid-lowering drugs), which can interfere with the body's natural store of CoQ10. Your medical practitioner may prescribe CoQ10 if you're taking such drugs. Again, I would suggest you keep your neurologist advised of the drugs you take and any supplements you choose to add.

We all have another naturally occurring antioxidant in our brain. It's called glutathione, and it may be depleted in Parkinson's disease. The role of glutathione is to protect the brain from damage by toxins. Some people with Parkinson's have reported benefits from treatment with intravenous glutathione, but there is no scientific proof to back these claims, and no proof that glutathione taken in this way could cross the blood–brain barrier to help where needed.

Magnesium

Magnesium strengthens our bones and helps maintain muscle and nerve function. Some people with Parkinson's believe it helps with sleeping and relieves the discomfort of restless legs. This is not proven, but it's relatively simple to maintain a good intake of magnesium, as it's found in green vegetables (particularly spinach), peas, beans, nuts, seeds and unrefined grains. Most of us meet our magnesium needs through a healthy diet.

The B vitamins

Folic acid is part of the B group complex which works to replenish neurotransmitters and replace nerve cells in the brain and nervous system. They are supposed to help improve memory. However, it's not recommended you take more than 50 mg of vitamin B6 daily as a supplement if you're on levodopa, as some research has shown B6 may block the effect of levodopa. It's best to get your B vitamins naturally in a variety of foods such as fish and seafood, whole grains, oatmeal, chicken, beef and eggs, leafy green vegetables, avocado, bananas, beans and peas, oranges, lemons and peanuts.

Vitamin B6 also aids the production of niacin (B3) from tryptophan, an essential amino acid (building block of protein) sourced only from food. In turn, niacin (B3) helps the body produce serotonin, which acts as a calming agent in the brain and has a key role in sleeping. If you're having trouble sleeping, combine B6 foods (such as potatoes, bananas, salmon, chicken, spinach, avocado, fish, brown rice and green peas) with those in which tryptophan naturally occurs (such as milk, turkey, whole grains, bananas and eggs). Since most tryptophan foods are high in protein, take them one hour on either side of your levodopa medication.

A cautious approach

I am always careful not to criticise any complementary therapies or supplements that other people with Parkinson's try. We know the mind benefit that can result from a placebo. However, make sure you research any complementary therapies, and check with your neurologist before using any supplements, as they may affect the efficacy of your medication. For example, you should not take a pharmaceutical tryptophan supplement or St John's wort (used to treat depression) if you are taking selective serotonin reuptake inhibitor drugs (SSRIs). As long as your neurologist or doctor knows what alternative healing you may be trying and has confirmed that it won't harm you, and as long as you can afford it, then you can go for it.

CHAPTER 15

⁂

Getting on with Parkinson's

I was standing in line in the bank when I noticed the man ahead of me. He wasn't outstandingly handsome, but was well dressed and attractive enough to get my attention. His hair was greying and he had a lined, intelligent face; he looked like he exercised at the gym and watched his weight, and he didn't seem to have any disability. I found myself thinking how much we're defined by our looks and our age. I wondered about the life he'd lived, what he'd done, the people he'd met and the story he held within. How much of the young man he once was did he still feel inside? And if he noticed me, what would he see? How do strangers perceive me? I'm sure Parkinson's has changed me, and yet I don't feel that different. When I got home I asked my husband if he ever noticed I had Parkinson's.

This was the first time I'd really thought about how others perceive us. Do we become someone who has Parkinson's? Do others see us as feeble, a bit crazy, or in need of help? Oh, I so hope not. Yet, in spite of the number of people with Parkinson's in the world, the condition is still little understood by those unaffected by it. Sometimes, if I notice someone looking at my shaking hand, I feel like saying, 'It's Parkinson's.' And at other times, when I'm poking around in my purse trying to get at the small change while others in the queue are sighing and looking impatient, I feel like saying, 'I've got Parkinson's and it slows me down.'

I have to say that as time has gone on, I have lost confidence. There are days when I do feel feeble and irrelevant. I can't think quickly enough, my voice is quiet; I shake too much and feel I have entirely lost my social skills. The more I feel like this, the more reduced I become. But then on other days I feel far from feeble. I can stride out, hold my head up and smile for all to see, and know that inside there still exists a confident, elegant, sexy and interesting woman.

Yet when meeting someone new who doesn't have Parkinson's, I feel sure that all they notice about me is the Parkinson's. It's tricky, because on the one hand I feel I should explain, but on the other hand I don't want them to think I'm a hypochondriac. Socialising has become more stressful than it should be. Being with family and friends is easier, as they've had time to grow used to any changes. So when my husband replied that he hardly ever noticed my tremor, dyskinesia or funny walk, I wasn't particularly surprised.

A summing up

I asked everyone who participated in this book to write down what they would say to someone newly diagnosed with Parkinson's, and most came back with similar replies. Their comments helped shape the content of this book. Here is a summary, as a quick reminder.

- ✦ First of all, don't panic.
- ✦ Take your time to come to terms with the diagnosis.
- ✦ Don't be in a rush to take medication unless you absolutely have to, but discuss this with your neurologist.
- ✦ You may not need medication for some time.
- ✦ Be responsible for your own experience of Parkinson's. Assess everything.
- ✦ Don't let Parkinson's define you.
- ✦ You don't have to stay with the first neurologist you see.
- ✦ Tell others about your diagnosis when you feel the time is right.
- ✦ Gather information when you're ready.
- ✦ Don't overdo the research to begin with.
- ✦ Join a Parkinson's organisation.
- ✦ Seek support only as you wish, and preferably from people of your own age.
- ✦ Your symptoms may be quite different from those of others.
- ✦ Keep exercising. If you'd already given up, join an exercise programme.

- Be aware that there are both physiological and psychological symptoms of Parkinson's.
- Get help if you're feeling depressed, stressed or anxious.
- Keep working for as long as you can.
- Seek professional medical, legal and financial advice, and plan for your future.
- Get legal advice about your employment contract. Anticipate possible problems before they happen.
- Ask questions. If you don't understand the answers, then ask again until you do.
- Write down the things that bother you.
- Remember there may be a settling-in period when you first go on medication.
- Keep a diary of how you feel on the medication during the settling-in period – for your eyes only.
- Don't put up with medication that's causing too many side effects without reporting it to your doctor.
- Your neurologist can help you understand why you may have to change medication at some stage.
- Trust your own judgement about how you're coping. It's your body; be responsible for it.
- Always check whether other drugs you take have any contra-indications with your Parkinson's medication.
- Make use of any complementary therapies within reason. Check with your neurologist or doctor first.
- Protect yourself with vaccinations, as Parkinson's lowers your immune system.
- Pace yourself and take time out to rest.
- Eat a healthy diet.
- Remain positive, and try not to give in.
- Recreate your life.
- Grab every opportunity to do something new.
- Be curious.
- Look on your condition as a reason to refocus on what's most important.
- Get lost sometimes – in other words, be daring enough to step outside your comfort zone.
- Don't become a stay-at-home wallflower – live life to the full.

What I wish

I wish well-meaning friends and strangers, those without Parkinson's, wouldn't say they'd just heard of a cure. When people first learn that you have Parkinson's, they often say things like: 'I read somewhere recently that they've discovered a new drug,' or, 'They're implanting stem cells now, aren't they?'

There is a great deal of research being done to find a cause and a cure for Parkinson's. I'd like this to happen in my lifetime, but who knows? I'm happy to donate my brain to a research programme, if it's of any use, so I guess that means I'm not holding my breath.

What I wish most of all is that by the time you've got to this part of the book you will have a better understanding of Parkinson's. I hope your family and friends will as well. Getting on with life is what it's about, and that means getting on with Parkinson's. I hope this book has helped you do just that.

BIBLIOGRAPHY

Ali, R. (2005) *I'll Hold Your Hand So You Won't Fall: A Child's Guide to Parkinson's Disease*. Merit Publishing.

BBC Horizon documentary (2001) 'Ecstasy and Agony', broadcast 15 February 2001.

Bradley, D. (2006) *Hyperventilation Syndrome: Breathing Pattern Disorders*. Random House.

Follet, K.A. et al. (2010) 'Pallidal versus subthalamic deep brain stimulation for Parkinson's disease.' *New England Journal of Medicine 362*, 2077–2091.

Fox, M. J. (2003) *Lucky Man: A Memoir*. Ebury Press.

Kaplitt, M.G. *et al.* (2007) 'Safety and tolerability of gene therapy with an adeno-associated virus (AAV) borne GAD gene for Parkinson's disease.' *Lancet 369*, 9579, 2097–2105.

Kübler-Ross, E. (2008) *On Death and Dying*. Routledge.

Langston, J.W. (1995) *The Case of the Frozen Addicts: Working at the Edge of the Mysteries of the Human Brain*. Pantheon Books.

Lewitt, P.A. *et al.* (2011) 'AAV2-GAD gene therapy for advanced Parkinson's disease: a double blind, sham surgery controlled, randomised trial.' *The Lancet Neurology*, Early Online Publication, 17 March 2011.

Lieberman, A. with McCall, M. (2003) *100 Questions & Answers about Parkinson's Disease*. Jones and Bartlett.

Luo, J. *et al.* (2002) 'Subthalamic GAD gene therapy in a Parkinson's disease rat model.' *Science 298*, 425–29.

Pollan, M. (2008) *In Defence of Food*. Allen Lane.

Roger, W. (1996) *Johnny Cash, Michael J Fox, John Walker… and Me*. Parkinson's New Zealand.

Sacks, O. (2008) *Musicophilia: Tales of Music and the Brain*. Picador.

Wallis, C. (2001) 'Surprising Clue to Parkinson's' in Time, 24 June 2001.

Woodward, D. (1999) 'Attitude and Exercise: Living with Parkinson's Disease', privately published booklet (available from woodpecker@kiwilink.co.nz).

USEFUL WEBSITES

Further support on Parkinson's

Parkinson's organisations provide education, information and support for all people with Parkinson's and for their caregivers, families and friends.

Australia: Parkinson's Australia www.parkinsons.org.au

New Zealand: Parkinson's New Zealand www.parkinsons.org.nz

United Kingdom: Parkinson's UK www.parkinsons.org.uk

United States: American Parkinson Disease Association www.apdaparkinson.org

American Parkinson Disease Association National Young Onset Center: www.youngparkinsons.org

Information about the brain

Centre for Brain Research, University of Auckland: www.fmhs.aukland.ac.nz/faculty/cbr

Neurological Foundation of New Zealand: www.neurological.org.nz

Neuroscience for Kids: http://faculty.washington.edu/chudler/neurok.html

Financial planning and budgeting

An independent money guide that offers New Zealand financial planning information and calculators: www.sorted.org.nz

GLOSSARY

AAV: Adeno-associated virus. A virus not associated with any human disease.

Acetylcholine: A chemical that works as a transmitter of nerve impulses in the brain, heart, stomach, bladder and peripheral nerves.

Agonist: A drug that enhances the activity of dopamine receptors.

Akathisia: *see* Restless legs.

Akinetic: Without tremor.

Alpha-synuclein: A protein of unknown function found in neural tissue; it clumps in the brain and kills neurons that produce dopamine.

Amantadine: A drug that helps release dopamine in the brain; originally designed to prevent influenza, it was later found to increase dopamine and suppress acetylcholine; marketed as Symmetrel.

Anticholinergic: Drugs that suppress acetylcholine; trihexyphenidyl (marketed as Artane) and benztropine (marketed as Cogentin).

Antioxidant: A substance that inhibits the destructive effect of free radicals in the body.

Anxiety: A state of stress.

Aspartame: An artificial sweetener; marketed as NutraSweet.

Ataxia: A problem with balance and walking.

Autonomic nervous system (ANS): Part of the brain and the nervous system that regulates the body's organs and glands.

Basal ganglia: A region of the brain encompassing the striatum, globus pallidus and thalamus.

Blastocyte: A fertilised egg.

Blood–brain barrier: Membrane that separates the blood from brain cells.

Bradykinesia: Slowness and loss of movement

Carbidopa: A drug that stops levodopa becoming dopamine before it reaches the brain.

Cerebral cortex: Layered neural tissue on the outer edge of the cerebrum which plays a key role in awareness, thought, language, memory, consciousness and attention.

Chondroitin: A sulphate which, along with glucosamine, supports the natural development of cartilage and helps mend connective tissue.

Chronic hyperventilation syndrome: A respiratory problem where the patient breathes shallowly and rapidly.

CR: Controlled-release (or slow-release) medication.

Deep brain stimulation (DBS): Surgery that involves implanting one or two electrodes into the damaged area of the brain, then attaching these to one or two pulse generators (stimulators) implanted in the upper chest area.

Depression: Chronic sadness.

DNA: Deoxyribonucleic acid. The molecule containing the genetic code of an organism.

Dopamine: A chemical produced by the brain that carries messages from one nerve cell to another (a neurotransmitter); too little dopamine in the motor areas of the brain is responsible for the symptoms of Parkinson's.

Dopaminergic neuron: A cell producing dopamine.

Dopamine agonist: A drug that stimulates dopamine receptors.

Dyskinesia: Involuntary jerky, twisting movements involving the whole body; a side effect of levodopa.

Dystonia: Involuntary muscle spasms that affect a single part of the body, such as the foot or even a toe; most likely, but not always, a side effect of levodopa.

Ecstasy: An illicit drug (MDMA).

Embryonic: Undeveloped.

Endorphin: Neurotransmitters that reduce pain.

Enteric nervous system: The nervous system controlling the bowels.

Essential tremor: A tremor disorder usually of the hands, head or voice, unrelated to Parkinson's; also called benign essential tremor.

Facial masking: A symptom of Parkinson's which immobilises face muscles.

Freezing: In Parkinson's, refers to moments when it becomes impossible to complete a movement.

GABA: An amino acid which acts as an inhibitory neurotransmitter and helps relaxation and sleep.

GAD: Glutamic acid decarboxylase. An enzyme necessary for the production of GABA.

Gene therapy: Inserting a healthy copy of a gene into a damaged area of the body.

Globus pallidus: Part of the basal ganglia affected by Parkinson's.

Glucosamine: A naturally occurring compound that repairs cartilage; can also be taken as a supplement, often with chondroitin.

Glutamate: An excitatory (stimulating) neurotransmitter that works in tandem with GABA, which is inhibitory (tranquillising); they are sometimes called the workhorses of the brain because of their stop–start roles.

Glutathione: A naturally existing antioxidant in the brain.

Hallucinations: The delusion that prompts someone to believe they have seen or heard something that does not exist.

Hemiplegic: On one side.

Hereditary: Passed on from parent to child.

Hypophonia: Soft voice.

Hypothalamus: An area in the brain that controls the autonomic nervous system (ANS) and the glands.

Idiopathic: Of unknown origin or apparent cause.

Kegel exercise: An exercise used to strengthen the muscles supporting the bladder.

Larynx: The portion of the respiratory tract that protects the voice box.

Lee Silverman Voice Treatment (LSVT): A system devised in USA for training a voice affected by Parkinson's.

Levodopa: A drug that converts into dopamine; sometimes referred to as L-dopa; marketed as Madopar and Sinemet.

Locked-in syndrome: A situation where a person is awake and aware, but unable to communicate.

Lumbar puncture: A procedure that involves inserting a needle into the spine and taking a sample of cerebrospinal fluid for testing.

Madopar: *see* Levodopa.

Micrographia: Small handwriting.

Mitochondria: The rod-like 'power plants' that sit within every cell and generate energy.

Monoamine oxidase B inhibitors: Parkinson's medications that prevent the breakdown of dopamine in the brain.

MPTP: An illicit narcotic known to cause instantaneous and incurable symptoms of Parkinson's.

MRI: Magnetic resonance imaging.

Multiple system atrophy (MSA): A condition similar to Parkinson's without tremor that does not respond to medication.

Neural plasticity: The ability of the brain to adapt to new conditions by forming new neural connections.

Neurologist: A doctor who specialises in diseases of the nervous system (brain, spinal cord, nerves).

Neurons: Nerve cells that process and transmit information in the brain.

Neuropathy: A form of nerve damage that may cause tingling, numbness or burning pain.

Neurotransmitters: Chemicals that transport impulses from one nerve cell to another; some of the most significant are acetylcholine, noradrenaline (norepinephrine), dopamine, serotonin, GABA, glutamate and endorphin.

Noradrenaline (norepinephrine): One of the neurotransmitters important to our sympathetic nervous system.

Olfactory bulb: Part of the nervous system that processes and transmits information received from cells in the nose to the brain.

Olfactory cortex: The area of the cerebrum that receives information and identifies odours.

Pallidotomy: An operation that destroys a small part of the globus pallidus.

Parkinsonism: A group of movement disorders including Parkinson's.

Pergolide: A dopamine receptor agonist.

Placebo: A simulated medical intervention, often a tablet containing no medication given to 50 per cent of participants in the medical trial of a new drug.

Pluripotent cells: Cells that can turn into any cell type in the body.

Postural hypotension: A drop in blood pressure when moving from one position to another – lying, sitting, standing.

Precursor cells: Cells used to encourage the pluripotent cells to develop into a particular type.

Progressive supranuclear palsy (PSP): Known as a PD+ ('Parkinson's Plus') disorder; distinguished from Parkinson's by its rapid onset of symptoms.

Restless legs: An aching discomfort that provokes the need to move the legs; the medical term is akathisia.

Retropulsion: A tendency to stagger or step backwards.

Ropinirole/Requip: An agonist that mimics the action of dopamine in the brain.

Selective serotonin reuptake inhibitor (SSRI): An antidepressant that increases the level of serotonin in the brain.

Serotonin: A neurotransmitter; along with dopamine it is sometimes called the 'feel good' chemical; loss of serotonin causes depression.

Sinemet: *see* Levodopa.

Speech difficulty: May be a slurring of speech and/or a loss of volume.

SSRI: *see* Selective serotonin reuptake inhibitor.

Statins: Drugs used to lower cholesterol levels.

Stem cells: Unspecialised cells that have the potential to develop into many different cell types.

Stevia: An artificial sweetener.

Substantia nigra: An area of the brain where cells produce dopamine; from the Latin, meaning 'black substance'.

Subthalamic nucleus: A small group of nerve cells about half the size of a peanut, situated close to the substantia nigra.

SWEDDs: Subjects without evidence of dopaminergic deficit; having a tremor of unknown origin with no other signs of Parkinson's and without loss of dopamine.

Symmetrel: *see* Amantadine.

Synapse: The gap between nerve cells across which impulses are relayed.

Thalamotomy: An operation that destroys a small area on one side of the thalamus in the brain.

Thalamus: A part of the brain that relays messages to and from every part of the brain, except the olfactory system.

Tremor: Often one of the first indications of Parkinson's; occurs initially on one side of the body when the hand is at rest.

Tryptophan: An essential amino acid not made by the brain, but acquired through food; it is the precursor to serotonin.

Vector: A virus modified to deliver genetic material to a cell.

Wearing off: Occurs when medications for Parkinson's slowly become ineffective.

Xylitol: An artificial sweetener.

INDEX